The Authentic HOMEMADE DOG FOOD COOKBOOK

Vet-Approved, Nutritious Allergy-Friendly Recipes for Dogs of All Sizes:

Feeding Guide, Storage Tips, PLUS Bonus Easy Slow Cooker Meals for Busy Dog Parents

DR. SAMANTHA REED

Paws & Plates Publishing

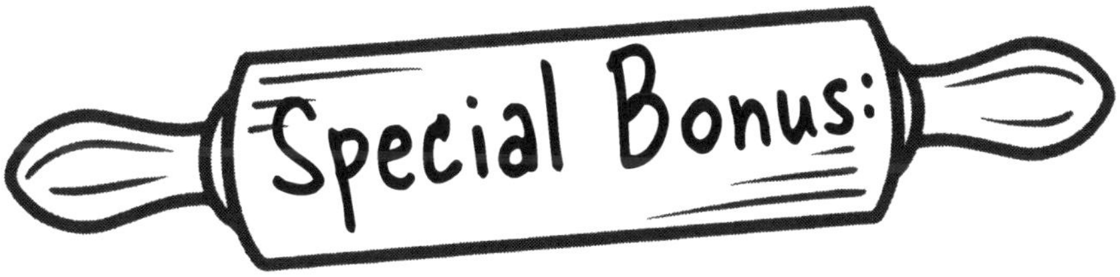

FREE RESOURCES TO HELP YOU MASTER HOMEMADE DOG NUTRITION

You're just one step away from enhancing your dog's nutrition and making mealtime stress-free!

As a special thank you for purchasing my homemade dog food book, I'm giving you **3 exclusive bonuses** designed to keep your pet happy and healthy, whether you're at home or on the go.

Simply go to https://geni.us/DogBookBonus or scan the QR code and access your bonuses today!

Bonuses You'll Receive:

- **Quick and Easy Slow Cooker Meals**
  Save time with these effortless, healthy meals your dog will love—perfect for busy days!
- **Healthy and Easy Homemade Dog Treats**
  Whip up nutritious treats with simple ingredients to keep your dog happy and healthy.
- **Healthy Eating While on The Go - Travel Guide**
  Never compromise on your pet's diet! Get tips for maintaining a healthy eating plan during travel.

TABLE OF CONTENTS

“Dogs are not our whole life, but they make our lives whole.”

—Roger Caras

INTRODUCTION

If you're reading this, it's because you're just as committed to your dog's health as I am. Welcome! When I first became a veterinarian, my mission was simple: to help animals live longer, healthier lives. Like many professionals, I trusted the conventional wisdom surrounding commercial pet foods and their promises of balanced nutrition. However, my entire perspective shifted when my own dog, Max, started experiencing mysterious health issues. Despite all my veterinary training and access to advanced treatments, nothing seemed to help. Max's health continued to decline, and I was left heartbroken and frustrated. I knew I had to do something different.

That's when I decided to look beyond traditional methods and focus on something fundamental: his diet. Switching Max from commercial pet food to homemade meals wasn't an easy decision, but it felt like my last hope. I started crafting meals from scratch, using fresh ingredients, carefully considering his nutritional needs, and making sure each meal was balanced. Slowly but surely, I saw changes—remarkable changes. His energy returned, his coat regained its natural shine, and, best of all, the playful, vibrant dog I had always known came back to life. This wasn't just a physical transformation—it was a profound reminder of the power of nutrition. I realized that a dog's diet isn't just important, it's critical for their health and longevity.

This personal journey with Max sparked a new passion in me: helping other pet owners understand the importance of what they feed their dogs. As a veterinarian, I had always emphasized nutrition to my clients, but seeing Max's recovery firsthand made me question the convenience and reliability of commercial pet foods. I became an advocate for homemade, balanced meals, because I saw the undeniable difference they made in a dog's health. And now, I want to share that knowledge and experience with you through this book.

What I have put together here isn't just a collection of recipes. It's a guide designed to empower you to take control of your dog's diet. You'll learn how to prepare nutritious, vet-approved meals using fresh ingredients that cater to your dog's specific needs—whether it's for weight management, digestive health, or simply overall well-being. And I know, transitioning to homemade meals can feel overwhelming. You might wonder, "Can I really do this?" or "What if I don't get the nutrition right?" or even "Will my dog like the food?" Rest assured, you're not alone. These are questions that so many pet owners have, and I'm here to guide you every step of the way.

In this book, we'll cover everything from the basics of canine nutrition to crafting easy, delicious recipes that you can prepare even on your busiest days. We'll break down the essential nutrients your dog needs, portion sizes, and how to tailor meals to your dog's unique health requirements. Whether you're a seasoned chef or someone who's never cooked a meal from scratch in your life, this book will make it simple and approachable for you to provide healthy, balanced meals for your dog.

And believe me when I say that homemade dog food doesn't have to be complicated or time-consuming. With just a few essential tools and some simple recipes, you'll soon see how easy it is to create meals that your dog will not only enjoy but will thrive on.

I've included practical tips, straightforward instructions, and recipes designed to be both nutritious and delicious. And don't worry, even if you're completely new to cooking, I've made sure these recipes are easy to follow and won't require hours in the kitchen.

Behind every recipe is my personal experience and expertise in veterinary dietetics. I've combined my scientific knowledge with my passion for animal health to create a resource that you can trust. Every meal and nutritional guideline in this book is backed by solid science and has been tested with real pets, my pets, ensuring you're providing the best possible care for your dog. My goal is to give you the confidence to make informed decisions about your dog's diet, knowing that you have the support of expert guidance along the way.

HOW TO USE THIS BOOK

Before we begin let me explain how I have created this book. It's divided into three key sections to make your transition to homemade dog food as seamless as possible. **In the first section**, we'll dive deep into the fundamentals of canine nutrition. Understanding what nutrients your dog needs and why they are important will equip you to make better decisions about their meals. We'll also dispel common myths about homemade pet food, giving you the tools you need to confidently create balanced, healthy meals for your dog.

In the second section, you'll find a variety of recipes tailored to meet your dog's individual needs. Whether you have a large breed, a small breed, a picky eater, or a dog with special dietary concerns, there's something for every pet. The recipes are easy to prepare with ingredients you can find at your local grocery store and are designed to provide balanced nutrition without overwhelming you.

Finally, **the third section** of the book presents a 30-day meal plan that simplifies the process of incorporating homemade meals into your dog's routine. This plan will help you maintain consistency while ensuring your dog gets all the nutrients they need. You'll also find shopping lists and practical checklists to help you stay organized and on track, making this journey as smooth as possible.

By making the switch to homemade dog food, you're not just changing what goes into your dog's bowl—you're making a significant impact on their overall health, happiness, and longevity. This book is your companion on that journey, providing the knowledge, recipes, and support you need to create a healthier life for your pet. Each meal you prepare brings you closer to a stronger bond with your dog, and contributes to a longer, happier life for them.

So, let's embark on this journey together. With every meal you make, you're giving your dog the best gift—better health and a better life. Here's to healthier, happier dogs and many more years of wagging tails!

Dr. Samantha Reed

CHAPTER 1: UNDERSTANDING DOG NUTRITION

Understanding dog nutrition is essential for ensuring your pet lives a healthy and happy life. Just like humans, dogs have specific dietary needs that change with age. Providing the right nutrients can significantly impact their energy levels, coat health, and overall well-being. It's not just about filling their bowls with food; it's about offering meals that support their growth, immune system, and longevity. Navigating canine nutrition can seem overwhelming, but knowing what to look for and how to balance their diet can simplify the process.

This chapter explores the core components of a dog's diet and the importance of each nutrient at different life stages. We'll cover the unique nutritional requirements for puppies, adults, and senior dogs, along with effective tips for meeting these needs. By the end of this chapter, my goal for you is that you will have the knowledge and basic understand of how you can boost up your dog's nutrition and improve their quality of life.

ESSENTIAL NUTRIENTS FOR CANINE HEALTH

Vital nutrients are the essential components that ensure a balanced diet for dogs and play critical roles in their overall health. Understanding these nutrients can help pet owners make informed decisions about their dog's nutrition. Let's explore the importance of proteins, fats, carbohydrates, vitamins, and minerals in your dog's diet.

The Importance of Proteins

Proteins are vital for muscle development, tissue repair, and immune function. They come from sources like lean meats, fish, and eggs, and should make up about 18-25% of a dog's daily caloric intake. The right protein level can vary based on age, health, and activity level. Foods rich in protein, such as chicken, beef, and fish, are highly digestible and provide essential amino acids needed for energy production and hormone regulation.

Not all proteins are equal however. Higher-quality animal proteins deliver a complete amino acid profile essential for your dog's health. For instance, chicken and beef are rich in protein and easy to digest. Additionally, fish like salmon provides high-quality protein and beneficial omega-3 fatty acids, promoting muscle health and a shiny coat.

Amino acids, which are the building blocks of proteins, are necessary for many bodily functions. Dogs need ten essential amino acids from their diet, as they cannot produce these on their own. Instead, they must be obtained from food. The ten essential amino acids for dogs include arginine, histidine, isoleucine, leucine, lysine, methionine, phenylalanine, threonine, tryptophan, and valine. Each of these plays a crucial role in various bodily functions. These amino acids support energy production and a functional immune system. Thus, a diet rich in various protein sources can help meet these needs. Don't worry though, the recipes covered in chapter 3 will help ensure your dog gets all ten.

The Role of Fats

Fats are a concentrated energy source and serve several important functions in a dog's health. They aid in absorbing fat-soluble vitamins (A, D, E, and K), promote healthy skin and coat, and are important for brain function. Fats should account for about 10-15% of a dog's diet, coming from fish oil, chicken fat, and flaxseed. These sources provide essential fatty acids, including omega-3 and omega-6, which help with your dogs cardiovascular health.

Balanced fat intake is crucial, particularly for active dogs that require higher energy levels. Fish oil is beneficial for delivering omega-3 fatty acids, known for reducing inflammation and promoting cognitive function. Where as chicken fat is a good source of omega-6 fatty acids that support skin health and a glossy coat.

Monitoring fat intake is important to prevent obesity, which can lead to health issues like joint problems and diabetes. It is essential to provide the right amount of fat in your dog's diet based on several key factors:

First, consider your dog's size. A small dog requires less fat compared to a large dog. For instance, a Chihuahua will need a different fat intake than a Labrador Retriever.

Second, take into account the breed of your dog. Certain breeds may have higher energy levels and metabolism, influencing their fat needs.

Lastly, consider their activity level. An active dog that runs and plays a lot will require more energy and thus may need a higher fat intake compared to a less active dog that enjoys lounging around the house.

Carbohydrates for Energy and Digestive Health

Carbohydrates provide energy and support digestive health for dogs. They can be sourced from whole grains, vegetables, and fruits, making up 30-50% of a dog's diet. Carbohydrates contribute essential fiber that promotes healthy digestion and regular bowel movements, especially benefiting physical activity.

Whole grains like brown rice and oats are great sources of carbohydrates, offering sustained energy and aiding gut health. Vegetables like sweet potatoes and peas provide carbohydrates along with vitamins and minerals, enhancing the overall diet. Fruits like apples and blueberries can be healthy treats, supplying antioxidants and dietary fiber.

Complex carbohydrates break down slowly, giving a steady release of energy and preventing blood sugar spikes. This slow digestion is ideal for maintaining consistent energy levels throughout the day, particularly for active or working dogs.

Vitamins and Minerals: Essential Nutrients

Vitamins and minerals are essential for various bodily functions, including metabolism, immune response, and bone development. These nutrients come from fruits, vegetables, and meats. Vitamins A, B, C, and E each have specific roles in maintaining health. For example, Vitamin A is important for vision and immune support, while Vitamin E serves as an antioxidant that protects cells from damage.

Minerals like calcium and phosphorus are crucial for strong bones and teeth. Iron is necessary for forming hemoglobin, which carries oxygen in the blood. A diet that includes a variety of fruits and vegetables can provide necessary vitamins and minerals. For instance, carrots are high in Vitamin A, while spinach includes iron and calcium.

Trace minerals like zinc and selenium, although needed in smaller amounts, are also important. Zinc supports skin health and wound healing, while selenium provides antioxidant protection against cell damage.

Incorporating a variety of nutrient-dense foods into your dog's diet can help fulfill their vitamin and mineral needs. Leafy greens, berries, carrots, and lean meats are excellent options to ensure your dog receives a broad range of essential nutrients.

NUTRITIONAL NEEDS FOR PUPPIES, ADULTS, AND SENIORS

Understanding the nutritional needs of dogs at different life stages is crucial to ensuring their health and well-being. Dogs, like people, have varying dietary requirements depending on their age. From the playful days of puppyhood, through the energetic adult years, and into the slower, more relaxed senior stage, each period demands specific nutritional attention.

Puppies

Puppies require a diet rich in protein and fat to support their rapid growth and boundless energy. These nutrients are vital as they develop muscle, bones, and internal organs. High-quality puppy food often contains around 22-32% protein and 10-25% fat, tailored to meet these needs. It's essential to choose foods that list animal-based proteins, such as chicken or beef, as the primary ingredient. This promotes healthy tissue development and overall growth.

For large breed puppies, it's critical to monitor calcium and phosphorus levels to prevent rapid bone growth that can lead to skeletal issues later in life. On the other hand, small breed puppies, with their higher metabolisms, might need more calorie-dense food. Feeding multiple small meals throughout the day can help manage their energy levels and prevent hypoglycemia.

Besides macronutrients, vitamins and minerals play a supportive role. For instance, DHA, an omega-3 fatty acid found in fish oil, aids in brain and vision development. Consistently providing a balanced diet from the start helps prevent developmental disorders and sets the foundation for a healthy adult dog.

Adult Dogs

Once a dog reaches adulthood, generally around one year for most breeds, their nutritional needs shift. Maintaining a balanced intake is key to supporting their health and new energy levels. Adult dogs typically need a diet lower in fat compared to puppies, usually around 9-15%. The protein requirement remains essential but slightly reduced, commonly at 18-25%.

The quality of protein continues to be important; lean meats, fish, and eggs are excellent sources. High-quality proteins help maintain muscle mass and ensure that the dog doesn't gain excess weight, which can lead to obesity and related health issues. Obesity in dogs can result in joint problems, diabetes, and heart disease.

Caloric intake should be adjusted based on the dog's activity level. Highly active dogs or working breeds may require more calories to sustain their energy needs. Conversely, more sedentary dogs benefit from a diet with fewer calories to prevent weight gain. Regular exercise complements proper nutrition in maintaining an ideal body weight and overall health.

Like I tell the owners who come into my clinic, that walk around the block is doing as much for your dog as it is for you. It's a win win!

Senior Dogs

Senior dogs, generally classified as those seven years and older, have unique nutritional needs. As their metabolism slows down, they require fewer calories to avoid weight gain. However, they still need nutrient-dense food to support their aging bodies.

Diets for senior dogs often include lower fat content, around 7-12%, while maintaining adequate protein levels to preserve muscle mass. Easily digestible nutrients become more important as their digestive systems may not work as efficiently. Ingredients like brown rice and sweet potatoes can be gentler on an older dog's stomach.

Increased fiber in a senior dog's diet aids digestion and helps manage weight. Joint health is another critical consideration; incorporating nutrients such as Omega-3 fatty acids from fish oil can reduce inflammation and support joint function. **Glucosamine and chondroitin supplements can also be beneficial for maintaining joint health and mobility**. I find this is often overlooked by a lot of my patients who have older dogs.

It's also essential to monitor for signs of cognitive decline in senior dogs. Antioxidants like vitamins E and C, as well as selenium, can support brain health. Always consult with a veterinarian to address specific health concerns and tailor the diet appropriately.

Life Stage Considerations

As dogs age, their nutrient needs shift, and being proactive about recognizing these changes is key to their health. Puppies need more frequent feeding schedules due to their high metabolism and smaller stomachs. Adults may thrive on two balanced meals a day. Seniors might benefit from smaller, more frequent meals to aid digestion and nutrient absorption.

Recognizing signs of nutritional deficiencies can encourage timely dietary adjustments. For example, a dull coat may indicate a lack of essential fatty acids, while lethargy could suggest inadequate protein intake. Monitoring weight, coat condition, energy levels, and stool quality provides valuable insights into whether their diet meets their current needs.

Transitioning your dog's diet appropriately at each life stage ensures they receive the right nutrients to thrive. Slow transitions between foods over a week can prevent gastrointestinal upset and allow the dog to adjust to new textures and flavors.

COMMON NUTRIENT DEFICIENCIES IN COMMERCIAL DOG FOOD

One common issue with commercial dog foods is their frequent lack of whole foods. Many of these products contain fillers such as corn, wheat, and soy instead of real food sources like meats, vegetables, and grains. These fillers may help to reduce costs for manufacturers, but they do not contribute much in terms of nutritional value for dogs. Instead, **commercial foods often rely on synthetic nutrients to meet the dietary**

requirements of pets. However, relying heavily on these synthetic additives can lead to nutrient imbalances over time. For instance, while vitamins and minerals are added to ensure complete nutrition, **the bioavailability of these nutrients — meaning how well an animal's body can absorb and use them — may not be as high as that from natural food sources**.

Another significant concern is essential **nutrient gaps found in many commercial dog foods**. Deficiencies in vitamins and minerals can have **serious long-term health implications for dogs**. For example, a diet lacking in vitamin A could lead to vision problems, while inadequate vitamin D intake may result in bone deformities or other skeletal issues. Omega-3 fatty acids are another crucial nutrient often insufficient in commercial diets. These fatty acids are vital for maintaining healthy skin and a shiny coat, as well as supporting brain and heart health. Dogs fed diets low in Omega-3s might show symptoms such as dry, flaky skin or a dull coat, indicating poor overall health.

Quality control in the pet food industry is another area where potential shortcomings can arise. Manufacturing practices can sometimes compromise the quality and safety of the food. Recalls due to contamination are more common than one might think. For example, microbiological contaminants like Salmonella and Listeria have been detected in some batches, posing health risks to both dogs and their owners (Kazimierska et al., 2021). Without stringent quality checks and adherence to safety standards, the risk of feeding contaminated food to pets remains high. This highlights the importance of staying informed about pet food recalls and understanding which brands have had quality control issues in the past.

Evaluating ingredients is a practice that all dog owners should master. Learning to read labels can make a significant difference in identifying high-quality foods versus those filled with unnecessary additives. **Ingredients are listed by weight, so ideally, meat or meat meal should be the first ingredient listed**. Fillers like corn, wheat, and soy indicate a less nutritious product. Additionally, terms like "by-products" can be misleading, as they may include parts of animals that are less desirable. By scrutinizing ingredient lists, owners can choose better options for their pets.

Understanding the nutritional adequacy statement on packaging is also crucial. This statement indicates whether the food meets the nutritional levels established by regulatory bodies. Foods labeled as "complete and balanced" have been formulated to provide all essential nutrients when fed according to the instructions on the label. However, it's always beneficial to look deeper into what constitutes "complete and balanced" in the context of your dog's specific needs. Factors such as age, breed, and activity level can influence these nutritional requirements significantly.

It's important to mention real-world examples of how these shortcomings manifest. For instance, a dog fed a diet primarily composed of low-quality commercial kibble may develop chronic conditions such as obesity, diabetes, or kidney disease. **Obesity in dogs is often related to high carbohydrate content in their diets, which can be traced back to those same fillers used in commercial foods**. Diabetes, similarly, can develop from prolonged consumption of high-sugar diets, again pointing to inferior commercial food quality.

SUPPLEMENTS

As a veterinarian, my mission has always been to help pets live their healthiest, happiest lives. Beyond providing a balanced diet, I've seen firsthand how the right supplements can make a profound difference in a dog's overall health. Supplements can address specific deficiencies and promote a range of benefits that regular dog food, including homemade alone may not fully cover.

The Role of Supplements

Even with the best diets, there can be gaps in nutrition that could impact your dog's long-term health. Supplements can bridge these gaps, supporting essential functions like immune health, joint maintenance, and digestive efficiency. In my practice, I've often recommended supplements to boost vitality, especially for dogs dealing with age-related concerns or specific health issues. When thoughtfully selected and carefully administered, supplements can work in harmony with your dog's diet to support overall longevity and vitality.

Common Types of Supplements

Multivitamins

Multivitamins are an excellent way to ensure your dog is getting a comprehensive range of essential vitamins and minerals. Even with a well-balanced diet, certain nutrients can be missed, especially as your dog ages or if they have specific dietary restrictions. These supplements typically include vitamins A, C, D, E, and B-complex, along with important minerals like calcium and zinc. They help to maintain energy levels, support the immune system, and promote overall health.

Joint Supplements

For dogs, especially older ones or those prone to joint issues, supplements like glucosamine, chondroitin, and collagen are invaluable. In my years of practice, I've seen these supplements significantly improve mobility and comfort in dogs suffering from arthritis or joint problems. Omega-3 fatty acids, usually sourced from fish oil, also support joint health by reducing inflammation and preserving cartilage. These supplements can help dogs dealing with conditions like osteoarthritis, allowing them to move with greater ease and less pain.

Probiotics

Gut health is critical to your dog's overall well-being. Probiotics, which are beneficial bacteria, help maintain a healthy digestive system. For dogs with gastrointestinal issues, probiotics can be particularly useful in improving nutrient absorption, boosting immune function, and even positively influencing mood and behavior. I often recommend probiotics for dogs that struggle with digestion or after they've been on antibiotics, as these can help restore healthy gut flora.

Consulting Your Veterinarian

Before introducing any supplement into your dog's routine, it's vital to consult with your veterinarian. Every dog has unique nutritional needs, and your vet can provide an individualized assessment based on factors like age, breed, weight, and any pre-existing health conditions. A professional evaluation ensures you're giving your dog the right supplements in the correct dosages, preventing unnecessary health risks.

Avoiding Health Risks

While supplements can greatly benefit your dog, they must be used properly. Over-supplementation can lead to serious health issues. For instance, too much vitamin D can result in kidney damage, while excessive calcium intake can cause skeletal abnormalities or urinary stones. This is why it's crucial to adhere to your vet's guidance and the dosing instructions on supplement packaging. Monitoring your dog for any adverse reactions is key to ensuring their continued safety.

Forms and Quality Control

Supplements come in various forms—powders, chewable tablets, liquids, and soft chews—making it easier to find something that suits your dog's preferences. Some dogs might prefer a flavored chew, while others may do better with a powder mixed into their food. However, no matter the form, the quality of the supplement is critical.

I always recommend choosing products that meet the quality standards set by organizations like the National Animal Supplement Council (NASC). This ensures the supplements you give your dog are both safe and effective. Pay close attention to labels and opt for brands with a solid reputation for transparency and efficacy.

A Holistic Approach to Health

I advocate for a holistic approach to your dog's health. While supplements can provide essential benefits, they are only one piece of the puzzle. A well-rounded approach includes a nutritious diet, regular exercise, hydration, and mental stimulation. Supplements should complement these practices, not replace them. Regular veterinary check-ups are also vital to ensure your dog's overall health is closely monitored and any potential issues are addressed early.

For a list of vet-approved supplements, turn to page 140.

CHAPTER 2: TRANSITIONING TO HOMEMADE DOG FOOD THE RIGHT WAY

Switching to homemade dog food can be a rewarding but careful process that greatly affects your dog's health. Knowing when your dog is ready for this change is important. Look for signs like changes in energy, digestive issues, unexpected weight changes, and increased dislike of certain foods to understand your dog's needs and readiness for a new diet. Paying attention to these signs helps ensure the transition meets their nutritional needs while keeping their digestion and overall health in check.

In this chapter, we'll look at how to tell if your dog is ready for a diet change. We'll discuss various signs to watch for, including behavioral changes and physical symptoms that indicate their current food may not be enough. By the end, you'll have a clear guide on when and how to introduce homemade meals for a smoother, healthier change for your dog.

IDENTIFYING SIGNS YOUR DOG IS READY FOR DIET CHANGE

Recognizing when your dog needs a new diet can make switching to homemade food easier. Being aware of the signs keeps your dog healthy during the change.

1. Changes in Energy Levels:

If your dog suddenly seems tired or overly energetic, their current food may not be right for them. A usually active dog that becomes sluggish might not be getting enough nutrients. On the other hand, a dog that is overly hyper could be reacting poorly to their commercial food. Monitoring your dog's energy throughout the day can help you determine if a dietary change is necessary. Matching their food to their activity level can help maintain their health.

2. Digestive Issues:

Digestive problems are another important sign. If your dog has bloating, gas, or irregular bowel movements, it might mean their current food isn't working well for them. Common signs include farting, stomach noises, or frequent diarrhea or constipation. These symptoms shouldn't be ignored, as they suggest that their diet may not suit their digestion. Switching to homemade food lets you know exactly what they're eating. Some dogs might also have sensitivities or allergies to ingredients in commercial foods, making homemade options better for them.

3. Unexplained Weight Changes:

Unexplained weight changes can indicate that your dog's diet isn't meeting their needs. If your dog is losing weight without a clear reason, they might not be getting enough calories or nutrition. Conversely, if they gain weight unexpectedly, their food may contain fillers that lead them to overeat. Weight fluctuations can also point to health issues like thyroid problems or diabetes, so it's a good idea to monitor their weight and consult a vet if there are significant changes. A balanced homemade diet can help stabilize their weight.

4. Changes in Appetite:

Keep an eye on your dog's appetite. If they seem less interested in their food or leave it in the bowl, it might be time for a change. This might be due to boredom with their diet or a negative reaction to certain ingredients. When dogs become picky, they can miss out on essential nutrients. Offering a variety of homemade meals can rekindle their interest in food and ensure they get a balanced diet. Pay attention to how they respond to different vegetables, proteins, and grains to create meals they enjoy.

5. Outside Factors:

Consider outside factors that could affect your dog's eating habits. Stressful events like moving or changes in routine can impact their appetite. Ensuring your dog feels safe and comfortable at mealtime can help them be more willing to try new foods. Gradually introducing homemade food in a calm environment can aid the transition.

Whenever you're thinking about changing your dog's diet, it's best to consult your veterinarian. They can provide tailored advice based on your dog's health history and needs, suggesting balanced recipes and portion sizes to ensure their new diet supports overall health.

STEP-BY-STEP TRANSITION PROCESS

Transitioning your dog from store-bought food to homemade meals can be a great experience for both of you, but it requires some planning to keep your dog's digestion and nutrition on track.

Start Gradually

Begin by slowly introducing homemade food into your dog's regular meals to avoid digestive issues. Mix a small amount of homemade food with their usual food—start with 20% homemade and 80% store-bought. Over the course of about a week, gradually increase the homemade portion until your dog is eating all homemade meals. This gradual change helps your dog adjust without stress.

Days	Homemade Food	Regular Food	Notes
1-4	25%	75%	Monitor for digestive upset: diarrhea, vomiting, gas, loss of appetite
5-8	50%	50%	Observe health and behavior, note any digestive issues
9-12	75%	25%	Check for adverse reactions: loose stools, stomach discomfort
13-16	100%	0%	Regular monitoring of health, watch for digestive problems

Keep a Journal

Track how your dog is reacting to the new food by keeping a journal. Record any changes in behavior, appetite, or health, and note signs such as increased energy, tiredness, vomiting, diarrhea, or changes in eating habits. This information helps you understand what works best for your dog and spot any potential problems early on. For example, if a certain ingredient causes issues, you can modify the recipe to avoid it.

Be Ready to Modify Recipes

Just like people, dogs have different tastes and may not tolerate all foods. Flexibility with your recipes allows you to meet your dog's needs, ensuring they enjoy their meals while getting proper nutrition. For example, if your dog is lactose intolerant, swap dairy for alternatives that won't upset their stomach.

Consult Your Vet Regularly

Check in with your vet during the transition. They can offer advice about your dog's nutritional needs, suggest changes to your recipes, and recommend supplements to ensure your dog is getting enough vitamins and minerals. If any issues arise during the switch, your vet can help troubleshoot.

Ensure a Balanced Diet

Maintaining a balanced diet is crucial when transitioning to homemade meals. Mix proteins, carbohydrates, and vegetables for a nutritious meal. Use meats like chicken or beef for protein, carbohydrates like rice or sweet potatoes for energy, and vegetables like carrots or peas for fiber and vitamins. Adjust your recipes based on your dog's age, weight, and activity level.

Monitor Weight

Weigh your dog regularly to ensure they are maintaining a healthy weight. Rapid changes in weight may indicate that the new diet isn't right for them. Monitoring their weight helps you make necessary adjustments. For recommendations be sure to check Vet Approved on page 139.

The following table shows normal weight ranges for various dog breeds:

Breed	Average Weight (lbs)	Average Weight (kg)
Beagle	20-30	9-14
Border Collie	27-45	12-20
Boxer	55-71	25-32
Chihuahua	3-6	1.5-3
Dachshund	16-32	7-14
French Bulldog	16-28	7-13
German Shepherd	50-90	23-41

Breed	Average Weight (lbs)	Average Weight (kg)
Golden Retriever	55-75	25-34
Great Dane	110-175	50-79
Labrador Retriever	55-80	25-36
Poodle (Standard)	45-70	20-32
Pug	14-18	6-8
Rottweiler	80-135	36-61
Shih Tzu	9-16	4-7
Siberian Husky	35-60	16-27
Staffordshire Bull Terrier	24-38	11-17
Yorkshire Terrier	4-7	2-3

Consider Smaller, More Frequent Meals

Instead of one or two large meals, consider smaller, more frequent feedings. This can aid digestion and reduce the risk of stomach upset. Your vet can help you determine the best feeding schedule and portion sizes for your dog's needs.

Incorporate Nutrient-Rich Ingredients

Include a range of nutrient-rich ingredients to boost your dog's health. For instance, adding eggs provides high-quality protein, while fish like salmon delivers healthy omega-3 fatty acids. Leafy greens aid digestion and support the immune system.

Introduce New Ingredients Slowly

When trying new ingredients, introduce them slowly and in small amounts. This allows you to identify any food sensitivities without causing digestive issues. Testing one ingredient at a time makes the transition smoother.

Stick to a Routine

Consistency is key to a smooth transition. Stick to regular meal times, portion sizes, and ingredients. A consistent feeding schedule can help prevent digestive problems and make tracking your dog's progress easier. This structure ensures your dog receives proper nutrition from their homemade meals.

MONITORING YOUR DOG'S RESPONSE TO NEW FOOD

This is part is key! Remember, switching your dog to homemade food can be a healthy change, but it's important to watch how they react. This will help keep your dog healthy and make sure they adjust well to the new diet. Here's what to look for.

Watch for Changes in Behavior

Keep an eye on your dog's energy and mood. If they seem more energetic or happy, that's a good sign. But if they seem tired or grumpy, something might be wrong. These changes can happen early, so it's important to notice them. A sudden change in behavior might mean the food isn't right for your dog.

Look for Physical Reactions

Watch for things like vomiting, diarrhea, or gas. Vomiting could mean your dog is having trouble with new ingredients, while diarrhea or gas could show that the food is too rich. If these problems keep happening, talk to your vet to see if the food needs adjustments.

Pay Attention to Eating Habits

How your dog eats can tell you a lot. If they eat with excitement, they probably like the new food. But if they eat less or take longer to finish, they might not like it or feel uncomfortable. Don't ignore this—it could mean the food isn't meeting their needs.

Adjust Recipes if Needed

Your dog may not like certain foods, or they may have trouble digesting them. If your dog has digestive issues, try adjusting the amount of protein, fats, or carbs. Introduce new ingredients one at a time, and watch how your dog responds.

Be Patient

The biggest tip I give my patients is switching to a new diet takes time and patience. Every dog is different, so what works for one dog may not work for another. Keep an eye on your dog, make changes as needed, and find what works best for them.

ADJUSTING PORTION SIZES DURING TRANSITION

Here's how to adjust portion sizes to avoid overfeeding or underfeeding during the switch.

First, take a look at your dog's current feeding routine. Find out how much commercial food your dog is eating now to set a baseline for changes. Measure the exact amount of kibble or wet food consumed daily. If you're estimating amounts, switch to a measuring cup or scale for accuracy. This helps you see your dog's current intake clearly, making it easier to figure out equivalent portions for homemade recipes.

Once you've established a baseline, gradually tweak the portions based on how your dog reacts to the new food. A sudden change can cause digestive issues like diarrhea or constipation. Instead, **slowly introduce the homemade food while reducing the old food** over several days or weeks, like in the chart I showed you earlier. Keep an eye on your dog for any signs of tummy trouble, such as vomiting, loose stools, or loss of appetite. If your dog seems uncomfortable, go slower with the transition. For example, if you're moving from 100% commercial food, start with 10% homemade food mixed with 90% commercial food and slowly increase the homemade portion every few days.

You may also want to **adjust the feeding schedule to offer smaller meals** more often throughout the day. Large meals can be hard on your dog's digestive system, especially when changing diets. Splitting the daily amount into three or four smaller meals can help digestion and provide steady nutrition. If your dog usually has two big meals, try dividing that into smaller portions. This can help maintain energy levels and lower the risk of bloating, especially for larger breeds.

It's also important to **know your dog's nutritional needs during this transition**. Puppies, for example, need more calories and nutrients than adult or senior dogs. Active dogs might require larger portions to match their energy uses, while less active dogs need fewer calories to avoid weight gain. Spayed or neutered dogs usually have lower metabolism and may need smaller portions than unaltered dogs.

Pay attention to the signs your dog shows during this change. **Keep track of their weight and condition regularly**. Weigh them at home using a pet scale or visit the vet's office. Track these weights to notice trends over time. The body condition score (BCS) ranges from 1 (emaciated) to 9 (obese), with the ideal score being around 4 to 5. You should be able to feel your dog's ribs without pressing hard and see a noticeable waist when you look down from above.

Avoid common mistakes like overfeeding treats or letting your dog free-feed during this time. **Treats shouldn't make up more than 10% of your dog's daily calories**. Choose healthy treats, like small veggie pieces, rather than calorie-dense store-bought options. And remember during this transition time, scheduled meals are better than free-feeding, as they help manage portions and create a consistent routine.

While your dog adjusts to homemade food, keep the ingredients and recipes consistent unless your vet advises otherwise. Sudden diet changes can upset your dog's stomach. If you want to try a new recipe, introduce it gradually by mixing it with the current food to help your dog's digestive system adjust smoothly.

Transitioning your dog to homemade food requires careful observation and gradual changes. The goal is to provide a balanced homemade diet that meets your dog's specific needs while maintaining their overall well-being. With patience and care, you can successfully transition your dog to a nutritious, homemade diet that enhances their health and happiness.

Now, lets get into the recipes!

CHAPTER 3: BALANCED NUTRITION FOR DOGS

In this chapter, you'll find a range of balanced recipes that have been the most popular ones with my patients over the years. It's important to give your dog the right nutrition, and we have recipes to fit every dietary need. Before we get into this I do want to cover the calcium to phosphorus ratio as well as the importance of multivitamins when feeding your dog homemade food.

Nutritional Sources Chart

Essential Nutrients	Food Sources
Lean Proteins	Chicken, Turkey, Beef, Fish, Lamb
Whole Grains	Brown Rice, Quinoa, Oats, Barley
Vegetables	Carrots, Spinach, Sweet Potatoes, Peas, Broccoli
Fruits	Blueberries, Apples, Bananas, Pumpkin, Watermelon
Healthy Fats	Fish Oil, Flaxseed Oil, Olive Oil
Dairy	Yogurt, Cottage Cheese (in moderation)
Herbs and Spices	Parsley, Turmeric, Ginger, Basil, Cilantro
Foods to Avoid	***Chocolate, Grapes, Onions, Garlic, Avocado***

This chart will help you quickly identify where to source the essential nutrients for your dog's diet, ensuring that you provide a well-rounded and healthy meal plan.

Understanding Nutritional Information

In each recipe, you'll notice percentages listed next to proteins, fats, and carbohydrates. These percentages represent the proportion of these macronutrients in the overall recipe and are intended as a guideline for balanced meals. The percentages do not add up to 100%, as they only reflect the macronutrient composition and not the total calories.

Adjusting Portions: You may adjust the serving size based on your dog's specific needs, weight, and activity level. For larger dogs, consider increasing portions, while smaller dogs may require less. If you're unsure, it's always a good idea to consult your veterinarian to determine the best portion sizes for your dog's nutritional needs.

How to Adjust the Calcium-to-Phosphorus Ratio in Your Dog's Recipes

Maintaining a proper **calcium-to-phosphorus ratio** is crucial for your dog's overall health, particularly for **bone development, muscle function, and metabolic processes**. Meat, which is naturally high in phosphorus, needs to be balanced with an appropriate source of calcium to prevent deficiencies.

For each recipe in this book, you can easily balance the phosphorus content by adding either **ground eggshells** or **bone meal** to the ingredients:

- **Ground eggshells**: A natural source of calcium, ground eggshells provide approximately **1,800-2,000 mg of calcium per teaspoon**. Adding **1/2 tsp** of ground eggshells per recipe with **4 oz of meat** will help ensure your dog's diet maintains a healthy balance.

- **Bone meal**: Bone meal offers both **calcium and phosphorus**, with a higher calcium content to help correct the ratio. Add **1/4 tsp of bone meal per 100g of meat** to your recipes for optimal results.

By making this simple adjustment, you'll be providing your dog with balanced nutrition in every meal.

Why You Need to Add a Multivitamin with Homemade Dog Food

When preparing homemade meals for your dog, it's important to understand the differences between **homemade food** and **commercial dog** food in terms of nutrient content. Commercially prepared dog foods are designed to meet specific nutritional standards, like those set by **AAFCO (Association of American Feed Control Officials)** and **FEDIAF (European Pet Food Industry Federation)**. These products are formulated to provide a complete and balanced diet, meaning all the necessary vitamins, minerals, and nutrients are already included.

However, when making food at home, you control the quality of the ingredients, but it's easy to miss out on essential nutrients like **vitamins A**, **D**, **E**, **calcium**, and **omega-3 fatty acids**. Even with high-quality ingredients, homemade recipes often fall short in providing a completely balanced diet. This is where a **multivitamin** becomes essential.

Why a Multivitamin Is Important for Homemade Meals:

1. **Balanced Nutrition**: Homemade meals can lack certain vitamins and minerals that are crucial for your dog's health. A multivitamin fills in these gaps, ensuring your dog gets everything they need in addition to fresh, high-quality ingredients.
2. **Joint and Digestive Support**: Many multivitamins include important supplements like **glucosamine** and **chondroitin** for joint health, as well as **digestive enzymes** and **probiotics** to support a healthy gut—nutrients that are harder to provide in a homemade diet.
3. **Vitamins A, D, and E**: These essential vitamins support a range of functions, from **immune health** to **bone strength** and **skin condition**. While certain foods provide these nutrients, it's often difficult to ensure your dog is getting enough in a homemade diet alone.
4. **Consistency**: Commercial dog foods are designed to be consistent in nutrient content, but homemade food can vary from meal to meal. Adding a multivitamin ensures that no matter what ingredients are used, your dog is getting a balanced and complete meal every time.

For these reasons, it's important to add a multivitamin with each meal. It's a simple step that makes sure your dog enjoys all the benefits of a homemade diet while maintaining the balanced nutrition they need for long-term health.

Check out Vet Approved on page 140 for the multivitamins that we recommend.

MEAT-BASED RECIPES

1. Beef & Brown Rice Bowl

Ingredients:

» 4 oz (113g) lean ground beef (cooked)

» 1/2 cup (90g) cooked brown rice

» 1/4 cup (30g) steamed carrots (diced)

» 1 tsp (5ml) olive oil

Nutritional Information:

» Final weight: 9.5 oz (270g)

» Calories: 320 kcal

» Proteins: 22%

» Fats: 15%

» Carbohydrates: 35%

Instructions:

5. Cook Beef: Sauté lean ground beef until cooked through, drain any excess fat.
6. Prepare Rice: Cook brown rice according to package instructions.
7. Steam Carrots: Steam or boil carrots until tender, dice into small pieces.
8. Combine Ingredients: Mix beef, rice, and carrots together.
9. Add Healthy Fats: Stir in olive oil and serve once cooled.

Ingredient Substitution Tips:

» Replace brown rice with oats for easier digestion.

» Swap carrots for peas for a different flavor profile.

Vitamins and Minerals:

» Iron: High (from beef)

» Fiber: Moderate (from rice and carrots)

» Vitamin A: Moderate (from carrots)

To meet AAFCO standards, we highly recommend adding a multivitamin to each meal. One of my favorite multivitamins that I recommend is this one.

https://amzn.to/3YpWSRI >>>

2. Lamb & Carrot Stew

Nutritional Information:

» Final weight: 9.5 oz (270g)

» Calories: 340 kcal

» Proteins: 20%

» Fats: 12%

» Carbohydrates: 35%

Ingredients:

» 4 oz (113g) lamb (cooked)

» 1/2 cup (90g) diced carrots (steamed)

» 1/4 cup (30g) cooked barley

» 1 tsp (5ml) olive oil

Instructions:

1. Cook Lamb: Brown the lamb in a pan until fully cooked.
2. Steam Carrots: Steam or boil the diced carrots until tender.
3. Combine Ingredients: Mix the cooked lamb, steamed carrots, and barley.
4. Add Healthy Fats: Drizzle olive oil over the mixture before serving.

Ingredient Substitution Tips:

» Replace barley with quinoa for added protein.

» Swap carrots with peas for a slightly sweeter dish.

Vitamins and Minerals:

» Protein: High (from lamb)

» Vitamin A: High (from carrots)

» Fiber: Moderate (from barley)

To meet AAFCO standards, we highly recommend adding a multivitamin to each meal. One of my favorite multivitamins that I recommend is this one.

https://amzn.to/3YpWSRl >>>

3. Pork & Apple Lunch

Ingredients:

» 4 oz (113g) cooked pork (lean cuts)

» 1/2 cup (90g) diced apples

» 1/4 cup (30g) cooked oats

» 1 tsp (5ml) flaxseed oil

Nutritional Information:

» Final weight: 9 oz (255g)

» Calories: 300 kcal

» Proteins: 22%

» Fats: 14%

» Carbohydrates: 30%

Instructions:

1. Cook Pork: Grill or boil the pork until fully cooked, then dice into small pieces.
2. Prepare Apples: Dice the apples into small pieces, leaving the skin on for fiber.
3. Cook Oats: Prepare the oats according to the package instructions.
4. Combine Ingredients: Mix pork, apples, and oats together in a bowl.
5. Add Healthy Fats: Drizzle flaxseed oil over the mixture before serving.

Ingredient Substitution Tips:

» Substitute apples with pears for a different flavor profile.

» Replace oats with brown rice for a more savory option.

Vitamins and Minerals:

» Fiber: High (from apples and oats)

» Protein: Moderate (from pork)

» Omega-3: Moderate (from flaxseed oil)

To meet AAFCO standards, we highly recommend adding a multivitamin to each meal. One of my favorite multivitamins that I recommend is this one.

https://amzn.to/3YpWSRI >>>

4. Beef Kidney & Quinoa Mix

Nutritional Information:

» Final weight: 9 oz (255g)

» Calories: 270 kcal

» Proteins: 25%

» Fats: 10%

» Carbohydrates: 35%

Ingredients:

» 4 oz (113g) beef kidney (boiled and chopped)

» 1/2 cup (90g) cooked quinoa

» 1/4 cup (30g) chopped green beans (steamed)

Instructions:

1. Boil Kidney: Boil beef kidney for 15-20 minutes until fully cooked, then chop into small pieces.
2. Cook Quinoa: Prepare quinoa according to package instructions.
3. Steam Green Beans: Steam green beans until tender and dice into small pieces.
4. Combine Ingredients: Mix beef kidney, quinoa, and green beans together.

Ingredient Substitution Tips:

» Replace beef kidney with liver for a different organ meat option.

» Use peas instead of green beans for variety.

Vitamins and Minerals:

» Iron: High (from beef kidney)

» Protein: High (from quinoa and beef kidney)

» Fiber: Moderate (from quinoa and green beans)

To meet AAFCO standards, we highly recommend adding a multivitamin to each meal. One of my favorite multivitamins that I recommend is this one.

https://amzn.to/3YpWSRl >>>

5. Venison & Carrot Blend

Nutritional Information:

» Final weight: 8.5 oz (240g)

» Calories: 320 kcal

» Proteins: 28%

» Fats: 12%

» Carbohydrates: 25%

Ingredients:

» 4 oz (113g) venison (cooked)

» 1/2 cup (90g) cooked carrots

» 1 tsp (5ml) coconut oil

Instructions:

1. Cook Venison: Grill or bake venison until fully cooked, then chop into small pieces.
2. Cook Carrots: Steam or boil carrots until tender, then dice into small pieces.
3. Combine Ingredients: Mix venison and carrots together in a bowl.
4. Add Healthy Fats: Drizzle coconut oil over the mixture before serving.

Ingredient Substitution Tips:

» Replace venison with lean beef for a more common protein.

» Substitute carrots with zucchini for a different vegetable option.

Vitamins and Minerals:

» Protein: High (from venison)

» Vitamin A: High (from carrots)

» Omega-6: Moderate (from coconut oil)

To meet AAFCO standards, we highly recommend adding a multivitamin to each meal. One of my favorite multivitamins that I recommend is this one.

https://amzn.to/3YpWSRI >>>

6. Lamb Kidney & Sweet Potato Mash

Nutritional Information:

» Final weight: 9 oz (255g)

» Calories: 290 kcal

» Proteins: 24%

» Fats: 10%

» Carbohydrates: 30%

Ingredients:

» 4 oz (113g) lamb kidney (cooked)

» 1/2 cup (90g) mashed sweet potatoes

» 1 tsp (5ml) flaxseed oil

Instructions:

1. Cook Lamb Kidney: Boil or bake lamb kidney until fully cooked, then chop into small pieces.
2. Prepare Sweet Potatoes: Boil sweet potatoes until tender, then mash them.
3. Combine Ingredients: Mix lamb kidney and mashed sweet potatoes.
4. Add Healthy Fats: Drizzle flaxseed oil and stir well.

Ingredient Substitution Tips:

» Replace lamb kidney with chicken liver for a lighter protein.

» Use pumpkin instead of sweet potato for a lower-calorie alternative.

Vitamins and Minerals:

» Protein: High (from lamb kidney)

» Vitamin A: High (from sweet potatoes)

» Omega-3: Moderate (from flaxseed oil)

To meet AAFCO standards, we highly recommend adding a multivitamin to each meal. One of my favorite multivitamins that I recommend is this one.

https://amzn.to/3YpWSRI >>>

7. Pork & Barley Stew

Nutritional Information:

» Final weight: 9 oz (255g)

» Calories: 310 kcal

» Proteins: 22%

» Fats: 12%

» Carbohydrates: 35%

Ingredients:

» 4 oz (113g) pork (cooked)

» 1/2 cup (90g) cooked barley

» 1/4 cup (30g) peas

» 1 tsp (5ml) olive oil

Instructions:

1. Cook Pork: Boil or grill the pork until fully cooked, then dice into small pieces.
2. Prepare Barley: Cook barley according to package instructions.
3. Cook Peas: Steam or boil peas until tender.
4. Combine Ingredients: Mix pork, barley, and peas together in a bowl.
5. Add Healthy Fats: Drizzle olive oil and stir well.

Ingredient Substitution Tips:

» Replace barley with oats for a softer grain.

» Use carrots instead of peas for a different flavor.

Vitamins and Minerals:

» Fiber: Moderate (from barley and peas)

» Protein: Moderate (from pork)

» Omega-3: Moderate (from olive oil)

To meet AAFCO standards, we highly recommend adding a multivitamin to each meal. One of my favorite multivitamins that I recommend is this one.

https://amzn.to/3YpWSRI >>>

8. Beef Liver & Pumpkin Mix

Ingredients:

» 4 oz (113g) beef liver (cooked)

» 1/2 cup (90g) cooked pumpkin (pureed)

» 1 tsp (5ml) coconut oil

Nutritional Information:

» Final weight: 8 oz (230g)

» Calories: 280 kcal

» Proteins: 22%

» Fats: 10%

» Carbohydrates: 25%

Instructions:

1. Cook Liver: Boil or grill beef liver until fully cooked, then chop into small pieces.
2. Prepare Pumpkin: Steam or bake pumpkin, then puree it until smooth.
3. Combine Ingredients: Mix liver and pumpkin puree together.
4. Add Healthy Fats: Drizzle coconut oil over the mixture before serving.

Ingredient Substitution Tips:

» Replace beef liver with chicken liver for a lighter option.

» Substitute pumpkin with sweet potatoes for a sweeter flavor.

Vitamins and Minerals:

» Protein: High (from liver)

» Vitamin A: High (from pumpkin)

» Omega-6: Moderate (from coconut oil)

To meet AAFCO standards, we highly recommend adding a multivitamin to each meal. One of my favorite multivitamins that I recommend is this one.

https://amzn.to/3YpWSRl >>>

9. Ground Beef & Zucchini Medley

Nutritional Information:

» Final weight: 9 oz (255g)

» Calories: 310 kcal

» Proteins: 22%

» Fats: 10%

» Carbohydrates: 35%

Ingredients:

» 4 oz (113g) ground beef (cooked)

» 1/2 cup (90g) chopped zucchini (steamed)

» 1/4 cup (30g) cooked brown rice

» 1 tsp (5ml) olive oil

Instructions:

1. Cook Ground Beef: Sauté ground beef until fully cooked, drain excess fat.
2. Prepare Zucchini: Steam or boil zucchini until tender, then chop.
3. Cook Rice: Prepare brown rice according to the package instructions.
4. Combine Ingredients: Mix beef, zucchini, and rice together in a bowl.
5. Add Healthy Fats: Drizzle olive oil over the mixture before serving.

Ingredient Substitution Tips:

» Replace brown rice with quinoa for extra protein.

» Use carrots instead of zucchini for a different texture.

Vitamins and Minerals:

» Iron: High (from beef)

» Fiber: Moderate (from rice and zucchini)

» Protein: High (from beef and rice)

To meet AAFCO standards, we highly recommend adding a multivitamin to each meal. One of my favorite multivitamins that I recommend is this one.

https://amzn.to/3YpWSRI >>>

10. Beef & Oats Breakfast Bowl

Nutritional Information:

» Final weight: 8.5 oz (240g)

» Calories: 290 kcal

» Proteins: 25%

» Fats: 12%

» Carbohydrates: 30%

Ingredients:

» 4 oz (113g) ground beef (cooked)

» 1/2 cup (90g) cooked oats

» 1 tsp (5ml) flaxseed oil

Instructions:

1. Cook Beef: Sauté ground beef until fully cooked.
2. Prepare Oats: Cook oats according to package instructions.
3. Combine Ingredients: Mix beef and oats together in a bowl.
4. Add Healthy Fats: Drizzle flaxseed oil over the mixture and stir well.

Ingredient Substitution Tips:

» Replace oats with barley for a chewier texture.

» Use chicken instead of beef for a leaner meal.

Vitamins and Minerals:

» Protein: High (from beef)

» Fiber: High (from oats)

» Omega-3: Moderate (from flaxseed oil)

To meet AAFCO standards, we highly recommend adding a multivitamin to each meal. One of my favorite multivitamins that I recommend is this one.

hhttps://amzn.to/3YpWSRI >>>

11. Pork & Oatmeal Breakfast

Ingredients:

» 4 oz (113g) cooked pork

» 1/2 cup (90g) cooked oats

» 1/4 cup (30g) diced apples

» 1 tsp (5ml) olive oil

Nutritional Information:

» Final weight: 9 oz (255g)

» Calories: 310 kcal

» Proteins: 22%

» Fats: 12%

» Carbohydrates: 35%

Instructions:

1. Cook Pork: Grill or boil pork until fully cooked, then dice into small pieces.
2. Prepare Oats: Cook oats according to package instructions.
3. Combine Ingredients: Mix pork, oats, and diced apples together in a bowl.
4. Add Healthy Fats: Drizzle olive oil over the mixture before serving.

Ingredient Substitution Tips:

» Replace apples with pears for a softer texture.

» Use quinoa instead of oats for a grain-free option.

Vitamins and Minerals:

» Protein: Moderate (from pork)

» Fiber: Moderate (from oats and apples)

» Omega-3: Moderate (from olive oil)

To meet AAFCO standards, we highly recommend adding a multivitamin to each meal. One of my favorite multivitamins that I recommend is this one.

https://amzn.to/3YpWSRI >>>

12. Beef Heart & Rice Mix

Ingredients:

» 4 oz (113g) beef heart (cooked)

» 1/2 cup (90g) cooked rice

» 1/4 cup (30g) peas

» 1 tsp (5ml) olive oil

Nutritional Information:

» Final weight: 9 oz (255g)

» Calories: 330 kcal

» Proteins: 28%

» Fats: 12%

» Carbohydrates: 35%

Instructions:

1. Cook Beef Heart: Boil or grill beef heart until fully cooked, then chop into small pieces.
2. Prepare Rice: Cook rice according to package instructions.
3. Cook Peas: Steam or boil peas until tender.
4. Combine Ingredients: Mix beef heart, rice, and peas together in a bowl.
5. Add Healthy Fats: Drizzle olive oil over the mixture before serving.

Ingredient Substitution Tips:

» Replace beef heart with liver for a different organ meat.

» Use sweet potatoes instead of rice for a different carbohydrate source.

Vitamins and Minerals:

» Iron: High (from beef heart)

» Protein: High (from beef heart and rice)

» Fiber: Moderate (from peas)

To meet AAFCO standards, we highly recommend adding a multivitamin to each meal. One of my favorite multivitamins that I recommend is this one.

https://amzn.to/3YpWSRl >>>

13. Venison & Sweet Potato Hash

Ingredients:

» 4 oz (113g) venison (cooked)

» 1/2 cup (90g) sweet potatoes (mashed)

» 1 tsp (5ml) olive oil

Nutritional Information:

» Final weight: 8.5 oz (240g)

» Calories: 300 kcal

» Proteins: 28%

» Fats: 10%

» Carbohydrates: 30%

Instructions:

1. Cook Venison: Grill or bake venison until fully cooked, then dice into small pieces.
2. Prepare Sweet Potatoes: Boil sweet potatoes until tender, then mash.
3. Combine Ingredients: Mix venison and mashed sweet potatoes together in a bowl.
4. Add Healthy Fats: Drizzle olive oil over the mixture and stir well.

Ingredient Substitution Tips:

» Replace venison with lean beef for a similar texture.

» Use pumpkin instead of sweet potatoes for a lower-calorie option.

TIPS

Vitamins and Minerals:

» Protein: High (from venison)

» Vitamin A: High (from sweet potatoes)

» Omega-3: Moderate (from olive oil)

To meet AAFCO standards, we highly recommend adding a multivitamin to each meal. One of my favorite multivitamins that I recommend is this one.

https://amzn.to/3YpWSRl >>>

14. Pork Liver & Barley Stew

Ingredients:

» 4 oz (113g) pork liver (cooked)

» 1/2 cup (90g) cooked barley

» 1/4 cup (30g) green beans (steamed)

» 1 tsp (5ml) coconut oil

Nutritional Information:

» Final weight: 9 oz (255g)

» Calories: 310 kcal

» Proteins: 25%

» Fats: 10%

» Carbohydrates: 30%

Instructions:

1. Cook Liver: Boil or grill pork liver until fully cooked, then chop into small pieces.
2. Prepare Barley: Cook barley according to package instructions.
3. Steam Green Beans: Steam green beans until tender, then chop.
4. Combine Ingredients: Mix pork liver, barley, and green beans together.
5. Add Healthy Fats: Drizzle coconut oil over the mixture before serving.

Ingredient Substitution Tips:

» Replace pork liver with chicken liver for a lighter option.

» Use carrots instead of green beans for a sweeter taste.

TIPS

Vitamins and Minerals:

» Protein: High (from liver)

» Fiber: Moderate (from barley and green beans)

» Omega-6: Moderate (from coconut oil)

To meet AAFCO standards, we highly recommend adding a multivitamin to each meal. One of my favorite multivitamins that I recommend is this one.

https://amzn.to/3YpWSRl >>>

15. Ground Beef & Sweet Potato Mix

Nutritional Information:

- » Final weight: 9 oz (255g)
- » Calories: 310 kcal
- » Proteins: 22%
- » Fats: 12%
- » Carbohydrates: 35%

Ingredients:

- » 4 oz (113g) ground beef (cooked)
- » 1/2 cup (90g) mashed sweet potatoes
- » 1/4 cup (30g) cooked peas
- » 1 tsp (5ml) flaxseed oil

Instructions:

1. Cook Ground Beef: Sauté ground beef until fully cooked, drain any excess fat.
2. Prepare Sweet Potatoes: Boil sweet potatoes until tender, then mash.
3. Cook Peas: Steam or boil peas until tender.
4. Combine Ingredients: Mix beef, mashed sweet potatoes, and peas together in a bowl.
5. Add Healthy Fats: Drizzle flaxseed oil over the mixture before serving.

Ingredient Substitution Tips:

- » Replace ground beef with turkey for a leaner option.
- » Use pumpkin instead of sweet potatoes for a lower-calorie alternative.

Vitamins and Minerals:

- » Protein: Moderate (from beef)
- » Vitamin A: High (from sweet potatoes)
- » Omega-3: Moderate (from flaxseed oil)

To meet AAFCO standards, we highly recommend adding a multivitamin to each meal. One of my favorite multivitamins that I recommend is this one.

https://amzn.to/3YpWSRl >>>

CHICKEN-BASED RECIPES

1. Chicken & Quinoa Power Bowl

Ingredients:

» 4 oz (113g) cooked chicken breast (skinless, boneless)

» 1/2 cup (90g) cooked quinoa

» 1/4 cup (30g) steamed broccoli (chopped)

» 1 tsp (5ml) olive oil

Nutritional Information:

» Final weight: 9 oz (255g)

» Calories: 300 kcal

» Proteins: 26%

» Fats: 10%

» Carbohydrates: 30%

Instructions:

1. Cook Chicken: Grill or boil the chicken breast until fully cooked, then dice into small pieces.
2. Cook Quinoa: Prepare quinoa according to package instructions.
3. Steam Broccoli: Steam broccoli until tender, then chop into small pieces.
4. Combine Ingredients: Mix the chicken, quinoa, and broccoli in a bowl.
5. Add Healthy Fats: Drizzle olive oil over the mixture before serving.

Ingredient Substitution Tips:

» Replace broccoli with spinach for a softer vegetable option.

» Use brown rice instead of quinoa for a different grain.

Vitamins and Minerals:

» Protein: High (from chicken and quinoa)

» Fiber: Moderate (from quinoa and broccoli)

» Omega-6: Moderate (from olive oil)

To meet AAFCO standards, we highly recommend adding a multivitamin to each meal. One of my favorite multivitamins that I recommend is this one.

https://amzn.to/3YpWSRI >>>

2. Chicken & Sweet Potato Mash

Ingredients:

» 4 oz (113g) cooked chicken breast (skinless, boneless)

» 1/2 cup (90g) mashed sweet potatoes

» 1/4 cup (30g) cooked peas

» 1 tsp (5ml) olive oil

Nutritional Information:

» Final weight: 9.5 oz (270g)

» Calories: 310 kcal

» Proteins: 24%

» Fats: 10%

» Carbohydrates: 30%

Instructions:

1. Cook Chicken: Grill or boil chicken breast until fully cooked and dice into small pieces.
2. Prepare Sweet Potatoes: Boil sweet potatoes until soft, then mash.
3. Cook Peas: Steam or boil peas until tender.
4. Combine Ingredients: Mix chicken, mashed sweet potatoes, and peas in a bowl.
5. Add Healthy Fats: Drizzle olive oil over the mixture before serving.

Ingredient Substitution Tips:

» Replace sweet potato with pumpkin for a different flavor.

» Substitute peas with green beans for variety.

Vitamins and Minerals:

» Protein: High (from chicken)

» Vitamin A: High (from sweet potatoes)

» Fiber: Moderate (from peas)

To meet AAFCO standards, we highly recommend adding a multivitamin to each meal. One of my favorite multivitamins that I recommend is this one.

https://amzn.to/3YpWSRl >>>

3. Chicken & Brown Rice Delight

Ingredients:

- » 4 oz (113g) cooked chicken breast (diced)
- » 1/2 cup (90g) cooked brown rice
- » 1/4 cup (30g) diced carrots (steamed)
- » 1 tsp (5ml) flaxseed oil

Nutritional Information:

- » Final weight: 9 oz (255g)
- » Calories: 300 kcal
- » Proteins: 25%
- » Fats: 10%
- » Carbohydrates: 35%

Instructions:

1. Cook Chicken: Boil or grill chicken until fully cooked, then dice.
2. Prepare Rice: Cook brown rice according to package instructions.
3. Cook Carrots: Steam or boil diced carrots until tender.
4. Combine Ingredients: Mix chicken, rice, and carrots in a bowl.
5. Add Healthy Fats: Stir in flaxseed oil.

Ingredient Substitution Tips:

- » Replace brown rice with quinoa for extra protein.
- » Use zucchini instead of carrots for variety.

Vitamins and Minerals:

- » Fiber: Moderate (from rice and carrots)
- » Protein: High (from chicken)
- » Omega-3: Moderate (from flaxseed oil)

4. Chicken & Pumpkin Bowl

Ingredients:

» 4 oz (113g) cooked chicken (diced)

» 1/2 cup (90g) cooked pumpkin (pureed)

» 1/4 cup (30g) cooked peas

» 1 tsp (5ml) olive oil

Nutritional Information:

» Final weight: 8.5 oz (240g)

» Calories: 280 kcal

» Proteins: 24%

» Fats: 10%

» Carbohydrates: 35%

Instructions:

1. Cook Chicken: Boil or grill chicken until fully cooked, then dice.
2. Prepare Pumpkin: Steam or bake pumpkin, then puree it until smooth.
3. Cook Peas: Steam or boil peas until tender.
4. Combine Ingredients: Mix chicken, pumpkin, and peas in a bowl.
5. Add Healthy Fats: Drizzle olive oil over the mixture.

Ingredient Substitution Tips:

» Replace pumpkin with sweet potatoes for a sweeter flavor.

» Use green beans instead of peas for variety.

Vitamins and Minerals:

» Protein: High (from chicken)

» Vitamin A: High (from pumpkin)

» Omega-3: Moderate (from olive oil)

To meet AAFCO standards, we highly recommend adding a multivitamin to each meal. One of my favorite multivitamins that I recommend is this one.

https://amzn.to/3YpWSRI >>>

5. Chicken & Oatmeal Breakfast

Nutritional Information:

- Final weight: 8 oz (225g)
- Calories: 290 kcal
- Proteins: 24%
- Fats: 12%
- Carbohydrates: 30%

Ingredients:

- 4 oz (113g) cooked chicken (diced)
- 1/2 cup (90g) cooked oats
- 1 tsp (5ml) flaxseed oil

Instructions:

1. Cook Chicken: Boil or grill chicken until fully cooked, then dice into small pieces.
2. Prepare Oats: Cook oats according to package instructions.
3. Combine Ingredients: Mix chicken and oats together in a bowl.
4. Add Healthy Fats: Stir in flaxseed oil before serving.

Ingredient Substitution Tips:

- Replace oats with brown rice for more texture.
- Use turkey instead of chicken for a different protein.

TIPS

Vitamins and Minerals:

- Fiber: High (from oats)
- Protein: Moderate (from chicken)
- Omega-3: Moderate (from flaxseed oil)

To meet AAFCO standards, we highly recommend adding a multivitamin to each meal. One of my favorite multivitamins that I recommend is this one.

https://amzn.to/3YpWSRl >>>

6. Chicken & Barley Stew

Nutritional Information:

- » Final weight: 9 oz (255g)
- » Calories: 300 kcal
- » Proteins: 24%
- » Fats: 10%
- » Carbohydrates: 35%

Ingredients:

- » 4 oz (113g) cooked chicken (diced)
- » 1/2 cup (90g) cooked barley
- » 1/4 cup (30g) diced carrots (steamed)
- » 1 tsp (5ml) olive oil

Instructions:

1. Cook Chicken: Grill or boil chicken until fully cooked, then dice.
2. Prepare Barley: Cook barley according to package instructions.
3. Cook Carrots: Steam or boil carrots until tender, then dice.
4. Combine Ingredients: Mix chicken, barley, and carrots in a bowl.
5. Add Healthy Fats: Stir in olive oil before serving.

Ingredient Substitution Tips:

- » Replace barley with quinoa for added protein.
- » Use green beans instead of carrots for variety.

Vitamins and Minerals:

- » Fiber: Moderate (from barley)
- » Protein: High (from chicken)
- » Vitamin A: High (from carrots)

To meet AAFCO standards, we highly recommend adding a multivitamin to each meal. One of my favorite multivitamins that I recommend is this one.

https://amzn.to/3YpWSRl >>>

7. Chicken Liver & Sweet Potato Mash

Nutritional Information:

» Final weight: 8.5 oz (240g)

» Calories: 280 kcal

» Proteins: 24%

» Fats: 12%

» Carbohydrates: 30%

Ingredients:

» 4 oz (113g) chicken liver (cooked)

» 1/2 cup (90g) mashed sweet potatoes

» 1/4 cup (30g) cooked peas

» 1 tsp (5ml) olive oil

Instructions:

1. Cook Chicken Liver: Boil or sauté chicken liver until fully cooked, then dice.
2. Prepare Sweet Potatoes: Boil sweet potatoes until soft, then mash.
3. Cook Peas: Steam or boil peas until tender.
4. Combine Ingredients: Mix chicken liver, mashed sweet potatoes, and peas together.
5. Add Healthy Fats: Drizzle olive oil before serving.

Ingredient Substitution Tips:

» Replace chicken liver with chicken breast for a lighter option.

» Use carrots instead of sweet potatoes for a different texture.

TIPS

Vitamins and Minerals:

» Iron: High (from chicken liver)

» Vitamin A: High (from sweet potatoes)

» Omega-6: Moderate (from olive oil)

To meet AAFCO standards, we highly recommend adding a multivitamin to each meal. One of my favorite multivitamins that I recommend is this one.

https://amzn.to/3YpWSRI >>>

8. Chicken & Carrot Blend

Ingredients:

» 4 oz (113g) cooked chicken breast (diced)

» 1/2 cup (90g) diced carrots (steamed)

» 1/4 cup (30g) cooked oats

» 1 tsp (5ml) flaxseed oil

Nutritional Information:

» Final weight: 9 oz (255g)

» Calories: 290 kcal

» Proteins: 24%

» Fats: 10%

» Carbohydrates: 35%

Instructions:

1. Cook Chicken: Boil or grill chicken until fully cooked, then dice.
2. Cook Carrots: Steam or boil carrots until tender, then dice.
3. Prepare Oats: Cook oats according to package instructions.
4. Combine Ingredients: Mix chicken, carrots, and oats in a bowl.
5. Add Healthy Fats: Stir in flaxseed oil.

Ingredient Substitution Tips:

» Replace oats with brown rice for a different texture.

» Use peas instead of carrots for a change in flavor.

TIPS

Vitamins and Minerals:

» Fiber: High (from oats and carrots)

» Protein: Moderate (from chicken)

» Omega-3: Moderate (from flaxseed oil)

To meet AAFCO standards, we highly recommend adding a multivitamin to each meal. One of my favorite multivitamins that I recommend is this one.

https://amzn.to/3YpWSRI >>>

9. Chicken & Spinach Stew

Nutritional Information:

» Final weight: 9 oz (255g)

» Calories: 290 kcal

» Proteins: 25%

» Fats: 10%

» Carbohydrates: 30%

Ingredients:

» 4 oz (113g) cooked chicken breast (diced)

» 1/2 cup (90g) steamed spinach

» 1/4 cup (30g) cooked quinoa

» 1 tsp (5ml) olive oil

Instructions:

1. Cook Chicken: Grill or boil chicken until fully cooked, then dice.
2. Steam Spinach: Lightly steam spinach until tender.
3. Cook Quinoa: Cook quinoa according to package instructions.
4. Combine Ingredients: Mix chicken, spinach, and quinoa together in a bowl.
5. Add Healthy Fats: Drizzle olive oil over the mixture before serving.

Ingredient Substitution Tips:

» Replace quinoa with barley for a different texture.

» Use kale instead of spinach for a slightly heartier meal.

Vitamins and Minerals:

» Protein: High (from chicken and quinoa)

» Iron: High (from spinach)

» Omega-3: Moderate (from olive oil)

To meet AAFCO standards, we highly recommend adding a multivitamin to each meal. One of my favorite multivitamins that I recommend is this one.

https://amzn.to/3YpWSRI >>>

10. Chicken & Kale Medley

Ingredients:

» 4 oz (113g) cooked chicken breast (diced)
» 1/2 cup (90g) steamed kale
» 1/4 cup (30g) cooked brown rice
» 1 tsp (5ml) olive oil

Nutritional Information:

» Final weight: 9 oz (255g)
» Calories: 300 kcal
» Proteins: 25%
» Fats: 10%
» Carbohydrates: 30%

Instructions:

1. Cook Chicken: Grill or boil chicken breast until fully cooked, then dice.
2. Steam Kale: Steam or boil kale until tender, then chop.
3. Prepare Rice: Cook brown rice according to package instructions.
4. Combine Ingredients: Mix chicken, kale, and brown rice together in a bowl.
5. Add Healthy Fats: Stir in olive oil before serving.

Ingredient Substitution Tips:

» Replace brown rice with oats for a lighter texture.
» Use spinach instead of kale for a milder flavor.

Vitamins and Minerals:

» Fiber: High (from rice and kale)
» Protein: High (from chicken)
» Omega-3: Moderate (from olive oil)

To meet AAFCO standards, we highly recommend adding a multivitamin to each meal. One of my favorite multivitamins that I recommend is this one.

https://amzn.to/3YpWSRI >>>

11. Chicken & Zucchini Medley

Ingredients:

» 4 oz (113g) cooked chicken breast (diced)

» 1/2 cup (90g) diced zucchini (steamed)

» 1/4 cup (30g) cooked barley

» 1 tsp (5ml) olive oil

Nutritional Information:

» Final weight: 9 oz (255g)

» Calories: 300 kcal

» Proteins: 25%

» Fats: 12%

» Carbohydrates: 30%

Instructions:

1. Cook Chicken: Grill or boil chicken breast until fully cooked, then dice.
2. Steam Zucchini: Lightly steam zucchini until tender.
3. Prepare Barley: Cook barley according to package instructions.
4. Combine Ingredients: Mix chicken, zucchini, and barley together in a bowl.
5. Add Healthy Fats: Drizzle olive oil over the mixture before serving.

Ingredient Substitution Tips:

» Replace zucchini with green beans for a different flavor.

» Use quinoa instead of barley for a lighter texture.

Vitamins and Minerals:

» Fiber: High (from barley and zucchini)

» Protein: High (from chicken)

» Omega-6: Moderate (from olive oil)

To meet AAFCO standards, we highly recommend adding a multivitamin to each meal. One of my favorite multivitamins that I recommend is this one.

https://amzn.to/3YpWSRl >>>

12. Chicken & Green Bean Blend

Ingredients:

» 4 oz (113g) cooked chicken breast (diced)

» 1/2 cup (90g) steamed green beans

» 1/4 cup (30g) cooked oats

» 1 tsp (5ml) flaxseed oil

Nutritional Information:

» Final weight: 9 oz (255g)

» Calories: 290 kcal

» Proteins: 24%

» Fats: 10%

» Carbohydrates: 30%

Instructions:

1. Cook Chicken: Grill or boil chicken breast until fully cooked, then dice.
2. Cook Green Beans: Steam or boil green beans until tender, then chop.
3. Prepare Oats: Cook oats according to package instructions.
4. Combine Ingredients: Mix chicken, green beans, and oats together in a bowl.
5. Add Healthy Fats: Drizzle flaxseed oil over the mixture before serving.

Ingredient Substitution Tips:

» Replace oats with barley for a different texture.

» Use carrots instead of green beans for a change in flavor.

Vitamins and Minerals:

» Fiber: Moderate (from oats and green beans)

» Protein: High (from chicken)

» Omega-3: Moderate (from flaxseed oil)

To meet AAFCO standards, we highly recommend adding a multivitamin to each meal. One of my favorite multivitamins that I recommend is this one.

https://amzn.to/3YpWSRl >>>

13. Chicken & Pea Stew

Ingredients:

» 4 oz (113g) cooked chicken breast (diced)

» 1/2 cup (90g) cooked peas

» 1/4 cup (30g) cooked brown rice

» 1 tsp (5ml) olive oil

Nutritional Information:

» Final weight: 9 oz (255g)

» Calories: 300 kcal

» Proteins: 25%

» Fats: 10%

» Carbohydrates: 35%

Instructions:

1. Cook Chicken: Boil or grill chicken until fully cooked, then dice.
2. Cook Peas: Steam or boil peas until tender.
3. Prepare Brown Rice: Cook brown rice according to package instructions.
4. Combine Ingredients: Mix chicken, peas, and brown rice together in a bowl.
5. Add Healthy Fats: Drizzle olive oil over the mixture before serving.

Ingredient Substitution Tips:

» Replace peas with green beans for a different vegetable.

» Use quinoa instead of brown rice for more protein.

Vitamins and Minerals:

» Fiber: Moderate (from brown rice and peas)

» Protein: High (from chicken)

» Omega-3: Moderate (from olive oil)

To meet AAFCO standards, we highly recommend adding a multivitamin to each meal. One of my favorite multivitamins that I recommend is this one.

https://amzn.to/3YpWSRI >>>

14. Chicken & Broccoli Medley

Nutritional Information:

» Final weight: 9 oz (255g)

» Calories: 280 kcal

» Proteins: 24%

» Fats: 10%

» Carbohydrates: 30%

Ingredients:

» 4 oz (113g) cooked chicken breast (diced)

» 1/2 cup (90g) steamed broccoli

» 1/4 cup (30g) cooked oats

» 1 tsp (5ml) flaxseed oil

Instructions:

1. Cook Chicken: Boil or grill chicken until fully cooked, then dice.
2. Steam Broccoli: Lightly steam broccoli until tender, then chop.
3. Prepare Oats: Cook oats according to package instructions.
4. Combine Ingredients: Mix chicken, broccoli, and oats together in a bowl.
5. Add Healthy Fats: Stir in flaxseed oil before serving.

Ingredient Substitution Tips:

» Replace oats with brown rice for a different grain.

» Use peas instead of broccoli for variety.

Vitamins and Minerals:

» Fiber: Moderate (from oats and broccoli)

» Protein: High (from chicken)

» Omega-3: Moderate (from flaxseed oil)

To meet AAFCO standards, we highly recommend adding a multivitamin to each meal. One of my favorite multivitamins that I recommend is this one.

https://amzn.to/3YpWSRl >>>

15. Chicken & Cauliflower Stew

Nutritional Information:

» Final weight: 9 oz (255g)

» Calories: 290 kcal

» Proteins: 25%

» Fats: 10%

» Carbohydrates: 30%

Ingredients:

» 4 oz (113g) cooked chicken breast (diced)

» 1/2 cup (90g) steamed cauliflower

» 1/4 cup (30g) cooked quinoa

» 1 tsp (5ml) olive oil

Instructions:

1. Cook Chicken: Boil or grill chicken breast until fully cooked, then dice.
2. Steam Cauliflower: Steam or boil cauliflower until tender, then chop.
3. Cook Quinoa: Cook quinoa according to package instructions.
4. Combine Ingredients: Mix chicken, cauliflower, and quinoa in a bowl.
5. Add Healthy Fats: Drizzle olive oil over the mixture before serving.

Ingredient Substitution Tips:

» Replace quinoa with barley for a different texture.

» Use carrots instead of cauliflower for a milder flavor.

Vitamins and Minerals:

» Fiber: Moderate (from quinoa and cauliflower)

» Protein: High (from chicken)

» Omega-3: Moderate (from olive oil)

To meet AAFCO standards, we highly recommend adding a multivitamin to each meal. One of my favorite multivitamins that I recommend is this one.

https://amzn.to/3YpWSRl >>>

TURKEY-BASED RECIPES

1. Turkey & Sweet Potato Hash

Nutritional Information:

» Final weight: 9 oz (255g)

» Calories: 290 kcal

» Proteins: 25%

» Fats: 10%

» Carbohydrates: 30%

Ingredients:

» 4 oz (113g) ground turkey (cooked)

» 1/2 cup (90g) mashed sweet potatoes

» 1/4 cup (30g) cooked peas

» 1 tsp (5ml) olive oil

Instructions:

1. Cook Turkey: Sauté ground turkey until fully cooked, breaking it into small pieces.
2. Prepare Sweet Potatoes: Boil sweet potatoes until tender, then mash.
3. Cook Peas: Steam or boil peas until soft.
4. Combine Ingredients: Mix turkey, sweet potatoes, and peas in a bowl.
5. Add Healthy Fats: Drizzle olive oil before serving.

Ingredient Substitution Tips:

» Replace sweet potatoes with pumpkin for a lower-calorie option.

» Use green beans instead of peas for variety.

TIPS

Vitamins and Minerals:

» Protein: High (from turkey)

» Vitamin A: High (from sweet potatoes)

» Omega-3: Moderate (from olive oil)

To meet AAFCO standards, we highly recommend adding a multivitamin to each meal. One of my favorite multivitamins that I recommend is this one.

https://amzn.to/3YpWSRl >>>

2. Turkey & Barley Stew

Ingredients:

- » 4 oz (113g) ground turkey (cooked)
- » 1/2 cup (90g) cooked barley
- » 1/4 cup (30g) diced carrots (steamed)
- » 1 tsp (5ml) flaxseed oil

Nutritional Information:

- » Final weight: 9.5 oz (270g)
- » Calories: 310 kcal
- » Proteins: 25%
- » Fats: 12%
- » Carbohydrates: 35%

Instructions:

1. Cook Turkey: Sauté ground turkey until fully cooked.
2. Prepare Barley: Cook barley according to package instructions.
3. Cook Carrots: Steam or boil carrots until tender, then dice.
4. Combine Ingredients: Mix turkey, barley, and carrots in a bowl.
5. Add Healthy Fats: Stir in flaxseed oil before serving.

Ingredient Substitution Tips:

- » Replace barley with quinoa for a grain-free option.
- » Use zucchini instead of carrots for a lighter texture.

Vitamins and Minerals:

- » Fiber: Moderate (from barley)
- » Protein: High (from turkey)
- » Omega-3: Moderate (from flaxseed oil)

To meet AAFCO standards, we highly recommend adding a multivitamin to each meal. One of my favorite multivitamins that I recommend is this one.

https://amzn.to/3YpWSRl >>>

3. Turkey & Spinach Scramble

Ingredients:

» 4 oz (113g) ground turkey (cooked)

» 1/2 cup (90g) steamed spinach

» 1/4 cup (30g) cooked oats

» 1 tsp (5ml) olive oil

Nutritional Information:

» Final weight: 9 oz (255g)

» Calories: 290 kcal

» Proteins: 25%

» Fats: 10%

» Carbohydrates: 30%

Instructions:

1. Cook Turkey: Sauté ground turkey until fully cooked.
2. Steam Spinach: Steam spinach until wilted.
3. Prepare Oats: Cook oats according to package instructions.
4. Combine Ingredients: Mix turkey, spinach, and oats in a bowl.
5. Add Healthy Fats: Stir in olive oil before serving.

Ingredient Substitution Tips:

» Replace oats with quinoa for a different grain texture.

» Use kale instead of spinach for a heartier meal.

TIPS

Vitamins and Minerals:

» Protein: High (from turkey)

» Iron: High (from spinach)

» Fiber: High (from oats)

To meet AAFCO standards, we highly recommend adding a multivitamin to each meal. One of my favorite multivitamins that I recommend is this one.

https://amzn.to/3YpWSRl >>>

4. Turkey & Pumpkin Mash

Ingredients:

» 4 oz (113g) ground turkey (cooked)

» 1/2 cup (90g) cooked pumpkin (pureed)

» 1/4 cup (30g) cooked peas

» 1 tsp (5ml) olive oil

Nutritional Information:

» Final weight: 9 oz (255g)

» Calories: 280 kcal

» Proteins: 24%

» Fats: 10%

» Carbohydrates: 35%

Instructions:

1. Cook Turkey: Sauté turkey until fully cooked.
2. Prepare Pumpkin: Cook pumpkin, then puree it.
3. Cook Peas: Steam or boil peas until tender.
4. Combine Ingredients: Mix turkey, pumpkin, and peas in a bowl.
5. Add Healthy Fats: Drizzle olive oil before serving.

Ingredient Substitution Tips:

» Replace pumpkin with sweet potatoes for a sweeter flavor.

» Use carrots instead of peas for a change in taste.

Vitamins and Minerals:

» Protein: High (from turkey)

» Vitamin A: High (from pumpkin)

» Omega-3: Moderate (from olive oil)

To meet AAFCO standards, we highly recommend adding a multivitamin to each meal. One of my favorite multivitamins that I recommend is this one.

https://amzn.to/3YpWSRl >>>

5. Turkey & Quinoa Breakfast Bowl

Nutritional Information:

» Final weight: 8 oz (225g)

» Calories: 290 kcal

» Proteins: 25%

» Fats: 10%

» Carbohydrates: 30%

Ingredients:

» 4 oz (113g) ground turkey (cooked)

» 1/2 cup (90g) cooked quinoa

» 1 tsp (5ml) flaxseed oil

Instructions:

1. Cook Turkey: Sauté turkey until fully cooked.
2. Prepare Quinoa: Cook quinoa according to package instructions.
3. Combine Ingredients: Mix turkey and quinoa in a bowl.
4. Add Healthy Fats: Stir in flaxseed oil before serving.

Ingredient Substitution Tips:

» Replace quinoa with barley for a heartier grain option.

» Use chicken instead of turkey for a lighter alternative.

Vitamins and Minerals:

» Protein: High (from turkey and quinoa)

» Omega-3: Moderate (from flaxseed oil)

» Iron: Moderate (from quinoa)

To meet AAFCO standards, we highly recommend adding a multivitamin to each meal. One of my favorite multivitamins that I recommend is this one.

https://amzn.to/3YpWSRI >>>

6. Turkey & Broccoli Stir-Fry

Ingredients:

» 4 oz (113g) ground turkey (cooked)

» 1/2 cup (90g) steamed broccoli

» 1/4 cup (30g) cooked oats

» 1 tsp (5ml) olive oil

Nutritional Information:

» Final weight: 9 oz (255g)

» Calories: 290 kcal

» Proteins: 25%

» Fats: 10%

» Carbohydrates: 35%

Instructions:

1. Cook Turkey: Sauté turkey until fully cooked.
2. Steam Broccoli: Lightly steam broccoli until tender, then chop.
3. Prepare Oats: Cook oats according to package instructions.
4. Combine Ingredients: Mix turkey, broccoli, and oats together in a bowl.
5. Add Healthy Fats: Drizzle olive oil over the mixture.

Ingredient Substitution Tips:

» Replace oats with brown rice for a more substantial grain.

» Use green beans instead of broccoli for variety.

Vitamins and Minerals:

» Fiber: Moderate (from oats and broccoli)

» Protein: High (from turkey)

» Omega-6: Moderate (from olive oil)

To meet AAFCO standards, we highly recommend adding a multivitamin to each meal. One of my favorite multivitamins that I recommend is this one.

https://amzn.to/3YpWSRl >>>

7. Turkey & Carrot Blend

Ingredients:

» 4 oz (113g) ground turkey (cooked)

» 1/2 cup (90g) diced carrots (steamed)

» 1/4 cup (30g) cooked brown rice

» 1 tsp (5ml) olive oil

Nutritional Information:

» Final weight: 9 oz (255g)

» Calories: 290 kcal

» Proteins: 25%

» Fats: 10%

» Carbohydrates: 35%

Instructions:

1. Cook Turkey: Sauté turkey until fully cooked.
2. Cook Carrots: Steam or boil carrots until tender.
3. Prepare Rice: Cook brown rice according to package instructions.
4. Combine Ingredients: Mix turkey, carrots, and brown rice in a bowl.
5. Add Healthy Fats: Drizzle olive oil over the mixture before serving.

Ingredient Substitution Tips:

» Replace brown rice with oats for a softer grain.

» Use zucchini instead of carrots for a different vegetable option.

Vitamins and Minerals:

» Fiber: Moderate (from brown rice and carrots)

» Protein: High (from turkey)

» Omega-6: Moderate (from olive oil)

To meet AAFCO standards, we highly recommend adding a multivitamin to each meal. One of my favorite multivitamins that I recommend is this one.

https://amzn.to/3YpWSRI >>>

8. Turkey & Pea Medley

Nutritional Information:

» Final weight: 9 oz (255g)

» Calories: 290 kcal

» Proteins: 25%

» Fats: 10%

» Carbohydrates: 35%

Ingredients:

» 4 oz (113g) ground turkey (cooked)

» 1/2 cup (90g) cooked peas

» 1/4 cup (30g) cooked oats

» 1 tsp (5ml) flaxseed oil

Instructions:

1. Cook Turkey: Sauté turkey until fully cooked.
2. Cook Peas: Steam or boil peas until tender.
3. Prepare Oats: Cook oats according to package instructions.
4. Combine Ingredients: Mix turkey, peas, and oats in a bowl.
5. Add Healthy Fats: Stir in flaxseed oil before serving.

Ingredient Substitution Tips:

» Replace oats with brown rice for a different grain.

» Use green beans instead of peas for a variety in vegetables.

Vitamins and Minerals:

» Fiber: Moderate (from peas and oats)

» Protein: High (from turkey)

» Omega-3: Moderate (from flaxseed oil)

To meet AAFCO standards, we highly recommend adding a multivitamin to each meal. One of my favorite multivitamins that I recommend is this one.

https://amzn.to/3YpWSRI >>>

9. Turkey & Zucchini Stew

Ingredients:

» 4 oz (113g) ground turkey (cooked)

» 1/2 cup (90g) steamed zucchini

» 1/4 cup (30g) cooked quinoa

» 1 tsp (5ml) olive oil

Nutritional Information:

» Final weight: 9 oz (255g)

» Calories: 290 kcal

» Proteins: 25%

» Fats: 10%

» Carbohydrates: 35%

Instructions:

1. Cook Turkey: Sauté turkey until fully cooked.
2. Steam Zucchini: Lightly steam zucchini until tender, then chop.
3. Prepare Quinoa: Cook quinoa according to package instructions.
4. Combine Ingredients: Mix turkey, zucchini, and quinoa together.
5. Add Healthy Fats: Drizzle olive oil over the mixture before serving.

Ingredient Substitution Tips:

» Replace quinoa with barley for a grainier texture.

» Use carrots instead of zucchini for a change in flavor.

Vitamins and Minerals:

» Fiber: Moderate (from zucchini and quinoa)

» Protein: High (from turkey)

» Omega-6: Moderate (from olive oil)

To meet AAFCO standards, we highly recommend adding a multivitamin to each meal. One of my favorite multivitamins that I recommend is this one.

https://amzn.to/3YpWSRI >>>

10. Turkey & Green Bean Bowl

Ingredients:

» 4 oz (113g) ground turkey (cooked)

» 1/2 cup (90g) steamed green beans

» 1/4 cup (30g) cooked oats

» 1 tsp (5ml) flaxseed oil

Nutritional Information:

» Final weight: 9 oz (255g)

» Calories: 290 kcal

» Proteins: 25%

» Fats: 10%

» Carbohydrates: 35%

Instructions:

1. Cook Turkey: Sauté turkey until fully cooked.
2. Steam Green Beans: Steam or boil green beans until tender, then chop.
3. Prepare Oats: Cook oats according to package instructions.
4. Combine Ingredients: Mix turkey, green beans, and oats in a bowl.
5. Add Healthy Fats: Stir in flaxseed oil before serving.

Ingredient Substitution Tips:

» Replace oats with barley for a different texture.

» Use carrots instead of green beans for more variety.

Vitamins and Minerals:

» Fiber: Moderate (from oats and green beans)

» Protein: High (from turkey)

» Omega-3: Moderate (from flaxseed oil)

To meet AAFCO standards, we highly recommend adding a multivitamin to each meal. One of my favorite multivitamins that I recommend is this one.

https://amzn.to/3YpWSRI >>>

FISH-BASED RECIPES

1. Salmon & Sweet Potato Mash

Nutritional Information:

» Final weight: 9 oz (255g)

» Calories: 310 kcal

» Proteins: 26%

» Fats: 12%

» Carbohydrates: 30%

Ingredients:

» 4 oz (113g) cooked salmon (boneless, skinless)

» 1/2 cup (90g) mashed sweet potatoes

» 1/4 cup (30g) cooked peas

» 1 tsp (5ml) olive oil

Instructions:

1. Cook Salmon: Bake or grill the salmon until fully cooked, then flake into small pieces.
2. Prepare Sweet Potatoes: Boil sweet potatoes until tender, then mash.
3. Cook Peas: Steam or boil peas until tender.
4. Combine Ingredients: Mix salmon, mashed sweet potatoes, and peas in a bowl.
5. Add Healthy Fats: Drizzle olive oil over the mixture before serving.

Ingredient Substitution Tips:

» Replace sweet potatoes with pumpkin for a different flavor.

» Use green beans instead of peas for a vegetable swap.

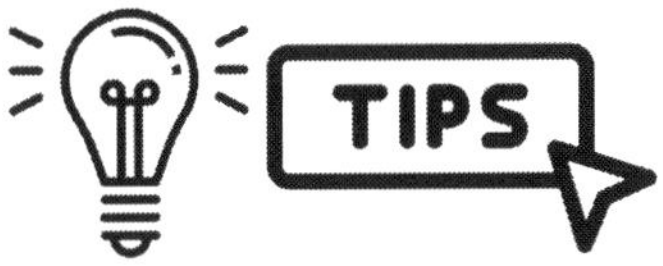

Vitamins and Minerals:

» Omega-3: High (from salmon)

» Vitamin A: High (from sweet potatoes)

» Protein: High (from salmon)

To meet AAFCO standards, we highly recommend adding a multivitamin to each meal. One of my favorite multivitamins that I recommend is this one.

https://amzn.to/3YpWSRl >>>

2. Cod & Carrot Blend

Ingredients:

» 4 oz (113g) cooked cod (boneless, skinless)

» 1/2 cup (90g) diced carrots (steamed)

» 1/4 cup (30g) cooked quinoa

» 1 tsp (5ml) flaxseed oil

Nutritional Information:

» Final weight: 9 oz (255g)

» Calories: 280 kcal

» Proteins: 24%

» Fats: 10%

» Carbohydrates: 30%

Instructions:

1. Cook Cod: Bake or grill cod until fully cooked, then flake into small pieces.
2. Cook Carrots: Steam or boil diced carrots until tender.
3. Prepare Quinoa: Cook quinoa according to package instructions.
4. Combine Ingredients: Mix cod, carrots, and quinoa in a bowl.
5. Add Healthy Fats: Drizzle flaxseed oil over the mixture before serving.

Ingredient Substitution Tips:

» Replace carrots with peas for a different vegetable profile.

» Use brown rice instead of quinoa for a change in grains.

Vitamins and Minerals:

» Omega-3: Moderate (from cod and flaxseed oil)

» Protein: High (from cod and quinoa)

» Vitamin A: Moderate (from carrots)

To meet AAFCO standards, we highly recommend adding a multivitamin to each meal. One of my favorite multivitamins that I recommend is this one.

https://amzn.to/3YpWSRl >>>

3. Tuna & Oatmeal Bowl

Nutritional Information:

» Final weight: 9 oz (255g)

» Calories: 290 kcal

» Proteins: 26%

» Fats: 12%

» Carbohydrates: 30%

Ingredients:

» 4 oz (113g) canned tuna (in water, drained)

» 1/2 cup (90g) cooked oats

» 1/4 cup (30g) diced zucchini (steamed)

» 1 tsp (5ml) olive oil

Instructions:

1. Prepare Tuna: Drain the canned tuna and flake into small pieces.
2. Prepare Oats: Cook oats according to package instructions.
3. Steam Zucchini: Lightly steam zucchini until tender, then dice.
4. Combine Ingredients: Mix tuna, oats, and zucchini in a bowl.
5. Add Healthy Fats: Drizzle olive oil over the mixture before serving.

Ingredient Substitution Tips:

TIPS

» Replace oats with quinoa for a protein boost.

» Use green beans instead of zucchini for variety.

Vitamins and Minerals:

» Omega-3: High (from tuna)

» Fiber: High (from oats)

» Protein: High (from tuna)

To meet AAFCO standards, we highly recommend adding a multivitamin to each meal. One of my favorite multivitamins that I recommend is this one.

https://amzn.to/3YpWSRI >>>

4. Sardine & Pea Salad

Ingredients:

» 4 oz (113g) sardines (boneless, skinless, in water)

» 1/2 cup (90g) cooked peas

» 1/4 cup (30g) cooked brown rice

» 1 tsp (5ml) olive oil

Nutritional Information:

» Final weight: 9 oz (255g)

» Calories: 280 kcal

» Proteins: 24%

» Fats: 12%

» Carbohydrates: 35%

Instructions:

1. Prepare Sardines: Drain sardines and flake into small pieces.
2. Cook Peas: Steam or boil peas until tender.
3. Prepare Brown Rice: Cook brown rice according to package instructions.
4. Combine Ingredients: Mix sardines, peas, and brown rice in a bowl.
5. Add Healthy Fats: Drizzle olive oil over the mixture before serving.

Ingredient Substitution Tips:

» Replace brown rice with barley for a different grain texture.

» Use carrots instead of peas for a sweeter vegetable.

Vitamins and Minerals:

» Omega-3: High (from sardines)

» Fiber: Moderate (from peas and brown rice)

» Protein: High (from sardines)

5. Mackerel & Sweet Potato Hash

Nutritional Information:

» Final weight: 9 oz (255g)

» Calories: 310 kcal

» Proteins: 26%

» Fats: 12%

» Carbohydrates: 30%

Ingredients:

» 4 oz (113g) cooked mackerel (boneless, skinless)

» 1/2 cup (90g) mashed sweet potatoes

» 1/4 cup (30g) steamed peas

» 1 tsp (5ml) flaxseed oil

Instructions:

1. Cook Mackerel: Bake or grill mackerel until fully cooked, then flake into small pieces.
2. Prepare Sweet Potatoes: Boil sweet potatoes until tender, then mash.
3. Cook Peas: Steam or boil peas until tender.
4. Combine Ingredients: Mix mackerel, mashed sweet potatoes, and peas in a bowl.
5. Add Healthy Fats: Drizzle flaxseed oil over the mixture before serving.

Ingredient Substitution Tips:

» Replace sweet potatoes with pumpkin for a lighter dish.

» Use green beans instead of peas for variety.

Vitamins and Minerals:

» Omega-3: High (from mackerel and flaxseed oil)

» Vitamin A: High (from sweet potatoes)

» Protein: High (from mackerel)

To meet AAFCO standards, we highly recommend adding a multivitamin to each meal. One of my favorite multivitamins that I recommend is this one.

https://amzn.to/3YpWSRI >>>

6. Salmon & Spinach Medley

Nutritional Information:

- » Final weight: 9 oz (255g)
- » Calories: 310 kcal
- » Proteins: 26%
- » Fats: 12%
- » Carbohydrates: 30%

Ingredients:

- » 4 oz (113g) cooked salmon (boneless, skinless)
- » 1/2 cup (90g) steamed spinach
- » 1/4 cup (30g) cooked quinoa
- » 1 tsp (5ml) olive oil

Instructions:

1. Cook Salmon: Bake or grill salmon until fully cooked, then flake into small pieces.
2. Steam Spinach: Steam spinach until wilted.
3. Cook Quinoa: Cook quinoa according to package instructions.
4. Combine Ingredients: Mix salmon, spinach, and quinoa in a bowl.
5. Add Healthy Fats: Drizzle olive oil over the mixture before serving.

Ingredient Substitution Tips:

- » Replace quinoa with brown rice for a heartier texture.
- » Use kale instead of spinach for a different leafy green.

Vitamins and Minerals:

- » Omega-3: High (from salmon)
- » Protein: High (from salmon and quinoa)
- » Iron: High (from spinach)

To meet AAFCO standards, we highly recommend adding a multivitamin to each meal. One of my favorite multivitamins that I recommend is this one.

https://amzn.to/3YpWSRI >>>

7. Tuna & Barley Stew

Ingredients:

» 4 oz (113g) canned tuna (in water, drained)

» 1/2 cup (90g) cooked barley

» 1/4 cup (30g) diced carrots (steamed)

» 1 tsp (5ml) flaxseed oil

Nutritional Information:

» Final weight: 9 oz (255g)

» Calories: 290 kcal

» Proteins: 26%

» Fats: 10%

» Carbohydrates: 35%

Instructions:

1. Prepare Tuna: Drain the tuna and flake into small pieces.
2. Cook Barley: Cook barley according to package instructions.
3. Cook Carrots: Steam or boil carrots until tender.
4. Combine Ingredients: Mix tuna, barley, and carrots in a bowl.
5. Add Healthy Fats: Stir in flaxseed oil before serving.

Ingredient Substitution Tips:

» Replace barley with oats for a different grain texture.

» Use green beans instead of carrots for a vegetable swap.

Vitamins and Minerals:

» Omega-3: High (from tuna)

» Protein: High (from tuna and barley)

» Vitamin A: High (from carrots)

To meet AAFCO standards, we highly recommend adding a multivitamin to each meal. One of my favorite multivitamins that I recommend is this one.

https://amzn.to/3YpWSRI >>>

8. Sardine & Quinoa Mix

Ingredients:

» 4 oz (113g) sardines (boneless, skinless, in water)

» 1/2 cup (90g) cooked quinoa

» 1/4 cup (30g) cooked peas

» 1 tsp (5ml) olive oil

Nutritional Information:

» Final weight: 9 oz (255g)

» Calories: 280 kcal

» Proteins: 24%

» Fats: 12%

» Carbohydrates: 35%

Instructions:

1. Prepare Sardines: Drain sardines and flake into small pieces.
2. Prepare Quinoa: Cook quinoa according to package instructions.
3. Cook Peas: Steam or boil peas until tender.
4. Combine Ingredients: Mix sardines, quinoa, and peas in a bowl.
5. Add Healthy Fats: Drizzle olive oil over the mixture before serving.

Ingredient Substitution Tips:

» Replace quinoa with brown rice for a different grain.

» Use carrots instead of peas for variety.

Vitamins and Minerals:

» Omega-3: High (from sardines)

» Fiber: Moderate (from quinoa and peas)

» Protein: High (from sardines)

To meet AAFCO standards, we highly recommend adding a multivitamin to each meal. One of my favorite multivitamins that I recommend is this one.

https://amzn.to/3YpWSRI >>>

9. Mackerel & Brown Rice Mix

Ingredients:

» 4 oz (113g) cooked mackerel (boneless, skinless)

» 1/2 cup (90g) cooked brown rice

» 1/4 cup (30g) cooked peas

» 1 tsp (5ml) flaxseed oil

Nutritional Information:

» Final weight: 9 oz (255g)

» Calories: 300 kcal

» Proteins: 26%

» Fats: 10%

» Carbohydrates: 35%

Instructions:

1. Cook Mackerel: Bake or grill mackerel until fully cooked, then flake into small pieces.
2. Prepare Brown Rice: Cook brown rice according to package instructions.
3. Cook Peas: Steam or boil peas until tender.
4. Combine Ingredients: Mix mackerel, brown rice, and peas in a bowl.
5. Add Healthy Fats: Stir in flaxseed oil before serving.

Ingredient Substitution Tips:

» Replace brown rice with quinoa for a different grain.

» Use zucchini instead of peas for more variety.

Vitamins and Minerals:

» Omega-3: High (from mackerel and flaxseed oil)

» Fiber: Moderate (from brown rice and peas)

» Protein: High (from mackerel)

To meet AAFCO standards, we highly recommend adding a multivitamin to each meal. One of my favorite multivitamins that I recommend is this one.

https://amzn.to/3YpWSRI >>>

10. Cod & Green Bean Medley

Nutritional Information:

- Final weight: 9 oz (255g)
- Calories: 280 kcal
- Proteins: 24%
- Fats: 10%
- Carbohydrates: 35%

Ingredients:

- 4 oz (113g) cooked cod (boneless, skinless)
- 1/2 cup (90g) steamed green beans
- 1/4 cup (30g) cooked quinoa
- 1 tsp (5ml) olive oil

Instructions:

1. Cook Cod: Bake or grill cod until fully cooked, then flake into small pieces.
2. Steam Green Beans: Lightly steam green beans until tender.
3. Prepare Quinoa: Cook quinoa according to package instructions.
4. Combine Ingredients: Mix cod, green beans, and quinoa in a bowl.
5. Add Healthy Fats: Drizzle olive oil over the mixture before serving.

Ingredient Substitution Tips:

- Replace quinoa with brown rice for a heartier texture.
- Use carrots instead of green beans for more variety.

Vitamins and Minerals:

- Omega-3: Moderate (from cod)
- Fiber: Moderate (from quinoa and green beans)
- Protein: High (from cod)

To meet AAFCO standards, we highly recommend adding a multivitamin to each meal. One of my favorite multivitamins that I recommend is this one.

https://amzn.to/3YpWSRI >>>

VEGETABLE-BASED RECIPES

1. Sweet Potato & Pea Mash

Ingredients:

» 1/2 cup (90g) mashed sweet potatoes

» 1/2 cup (90g) cooked peas

» 1 tsp (5ml) flaxseed oil

Nutritional Information:

» Final weight: 8.5 oz (240g)

» Calories: 180 kcal

» Proteins: 6%

» Fats: 8%

» Carbohydrates: 40%

Instructions:

1. Prepare Sweet Potatoes: Boil sweet potatoes until tender, then mash.
2. Cook Peas: Steam or boil peas until soft.
3. Combine Ingredients: Mix mashed sweet potatoes and peas in a bowl.
4. Add Healthy Fats: Stir in flaxseed oil before serving.

Ingredient Substitution Tips:

» Replace sweet potatoes with pumpkin for a different flavor.

» Use carrots instead of peas for a sweeter dish.

Vitamins and Minerals:

» Vitamin A: High (from sweet potatoes)

» Fiber: Moderate (from peas)

» Omega-3: Moderate (from flaxseed oil)

To meet AAFCO standards, we highly recommend adding a multivitamin to each meal. One of my favorite multivitamins that I recommend is this one.

https://amzn.to/3YpWSRI >>>

2. Carrot & Zucchini Blend

Nutritional Information:

» Final weight: 8 oz (230g)

» Calories: 120 kcal

» Proteins: 4%

» Fats: 8%

» Carbohydrates: 30%

Ingredients:

» 1/2 cup (90g) diced carrots (steamed)

» 1/2 cup (90g) steamed zucchini

» 1 tsp (5ml) olive oil

Instructions:

1. Cook Carrots: Steam or boil diced carrots until tender.
2. Steam Zucchini: Lightly steam zucchini until tender, then dice.
3. Combine Ingredients: Mix carrots and zucchini together in a bowl.
4. Add Healthy Fats: Drizzle olive oil over the mixture before serving.

Ingredient Substitution Tips:

» Replace carrots with sweet potatoes for a heartier dish.

» Use spinach instead of zucchini for a leafy green option.

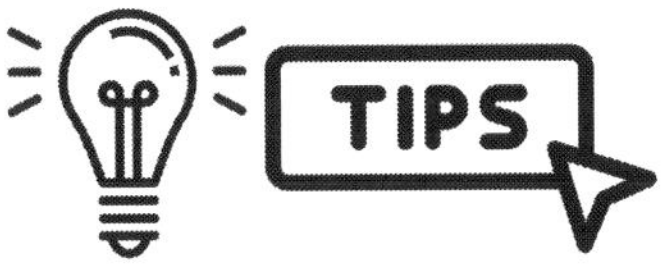

Vitamins and Minerals:

» Vitamin A: High (from carrots)

» Fiber: Moderate (from zucchini)

» Omega-6: Moderate (from olive oil)

To meet AAFCO standards, we highly recommend adding a multivitamin to each meal. One of my favorite multivitamins that I recommend is this one.

https://amzn.to/3YpWSRI >>>

3. Spinach & Sweet Potato Medley

Nutritional Information:

- » Final weight: 8 oz (230g)
- » Calories: 150 kcal
- » Proteins: 6%
- » Fats: 8%
- » Carbohydrates: 35%

Ingredients:

- » 1/2 cup (90g) steamed spinach
- » 1/2 cup (90g) mashed sweet potatoes
- » 1 tsp (5ml) olive oil

Instructions:

1. Steam Spinach: Steam spinach until wilted.
2. Prepare Sweet Potatoes: Boil sweet potatoes until tender, then mash.
3. Combine Ingredients: Mix spinach and sweet potatoes in a bowl.
4. Add Healthy Fats: Stir in olive oil before serving.

Ingredient Substitution Tips:

- » Replace sweet potatoes with pumpkin for a lower-calorie option.
- » Use kale instead of spinach for a heartier dish.

Vitamins and Minerals:

- » Vitamin A: High (from sweet potatoes and spinach)
- » Iron: High (from spinach)
- » Omega-6: Moderate (from olive oil)

To meet AAFCO standards, we highly recommend adding a multivitamin to each meal. One of my favorite multivitamins that I recommend is this one.

https://amzn.to/3YpWSRI >>>

4. Pumpkin & Carrot Bowl

Nutritional Information:

» Final weight: 8 oz (230g)

» Calories: 140 kcal

» Proteins: 5%

» Fats: 8%

» Carbohydrates: 35%

Ingredients:

» 1/2 cup (90g) cooked pumpkin (pureed)

» 1/2 cup (90g) diced carrots (steamed)

» 1 tsp (5ml) flaxseed oil

Instructions:

1. Prepare Pumpkin: Steam or bake pumpkin, then puree it.
2. Cook Carrots: Steam or boil diced carrots until tender.
3. Combine Ingredients: Mix pumpkin and carrots in a bowl.
4. Add Healthy Fats: Stir in flaxseed oil before serving.

Ingredient Substitution Tips:

» Replace pumpkin with sweet potatoes for a denser texture.

» Use zucchini instead of carrots for variety.

TIPS

Vitamins and Minerals:

» Vitamin A: High (from pumpkin and carrots)

» Fiber: Moderate (from carrots)

» Omega-3: Moderate (from flaxseed oil)

To meet AAFCO standards, we highly recommend adding a multivitamin to each meal. One of my favorite multivitamins that I recommend is this one.

https://amzn.to/3YpWSRI >>>

5. Green Bean & Sweet Potato Mash

Nutritional Information:

- » Final weight: 8 oz (230g)
- » Calories: 160 kcal
- » Proteins: 5%
- » Fats: 8%
- » Carbohydrates: 35%

Ingredients:

- » 1/2 cup (90g) mashed sweet potatoes
- » 1/2 cup (90g) steamed green beans
- » 1 tsp (5ml) olive oil

Instructions:

1. Prepare Sweet Potatoes: Boil sweet potatoes until tender, then mash.
2. Cook Green Beans: Steam or boil green beans until tender, then chop.
3. Combine Ingredients: Mix mashed sweet potatoes and green beans in a bowl.
4. Add Healthy Fats: Drizzle olive oil over the mixture before serving.

Ingredient Substitution Tips:

- » Replace sweet potatoes with pumpkin for a lower-calorie dish.
- » Use carrots instead of green beans for a different flavor profile.

Vitamins and Minerals:

- » Vitamin A: High (from sweet potatoes)
- » Fiber: Moderate (from green beans)
- » Omega-6: Moderate (from olive oil)

To meet AAFCO standards, we highly recommend adding a multivitamin to each meal. One of my favorite multivitamins that I recommend is this one.

https://amzn.to/3YpWSRI >>>

6. Kale & Carrot Blend

Nutritional Information:

» Final weight: 8 oz (230g)

» Calories: 130 kcal

» Proteins: 6%

» Fats: 8%

» Carbohydrates: 30%

Ingredients:

» 1/2 cup (90g) steamed kale

» 1/2 cup (90g) diced carrots (steamed)

» 1 tsp (5ml) olive oil

Instructions:

1. Steam Kale: Steam kale until wilted.
2. Cook Carrots: Steam or boil diced carrots until tender.
3. Combine Ingredients: Mix kale and carrots in a bowl.
4. Add Healthy Fats: Drizzle olive oil over the mixture before serving.

Ingredient Substitution Tips:

» Replace carrots with sweet potatoes for a different texture.

» Use spinach instead of kale for a lighter option.

Vitamins and Minerals:

» Iron: High (from kale)

» Vitamin A: High (from carrots)

» Omega-6: Moderate (from olive oil)

To meet AAFCO standards, we highly recommend adding a multivitamin to each meal. One of my favorite multivitamins that I recommend is this one.

https://amzn.to/3YpWSRI >>>

7. Broccoli & Pumpkin Mix

Ingredients:

» 1/2 cup (90g) steamed broccoli

» 1/2 cup (90g) cooked pumpkin (pureed)

» 1 tsp (5ml) flaxseed oil

Nutritional Information:

» Final weight: 8 oz (230g)

» Calories: 140 kcal

» Proteins: 5%

» Fats: 8%

» Carbohydrates: 30%

Instructions:

1. Steam Broccoli: Lightly steam broccoli until tender.
2. Prepare Pumpkin: Steam or bake pumpkin, then puree it.
3. Combine Ingredients: Mix broccoli and pumpkin in a bowl.
4. Add Healthy Fats: Stir in flaxseed oil before serving.

Ingredient Substitution Tips:

» Replace pumpkin with sweet potatoes for a denser mash.

» Use zucchini instead of broccoli for variety.

Vitamins and Minerals:

» Fiber: Moderate (from broccoli)

» Vitamin A: High (from pumpkin)

» Omega-3: Moderate (from flaxseed oil)

To meet AAFCO standards, we highly recommend adding a multivitamin to each meal. One of my favorite multivitamins that I recommend is this one.

https://amzn.to/3YpWSRI >>>

8. Zucchini & Spinach Bowl

Ingredients:

» 1/2 cup (90g) steamed zucchini

» 1/2 cup (90g) steamed spinach

» 1 tsp (5ml) olive oil

Nutritional Information:

» Final weight: 8 oz (230g)

» Calories: 120 kcal

» Proteins: 6%

» Fats: 8%

» Carbohydrates: 30%

Instructions:

1. Steam Zucchini: Lightly steam zucchini until tender, then dice.
2. Steam Spinach: Steam spinach until wilted.
3. Combine Ingredients: Mix zucchini and spinach in a bowl.
4. Add Healthy Fats: Drizzle olive oil over the mixture before serving.

Ingredient Substitution Tips:

» Replace spinach with kale for a heartier meal.

» Use peas instead of zucchini for a different vegetable.

TIPS

Vitamins and Minerals:

» Iron: High (from spinach)

» Fiber: Moderate (from zucchini)

» Omega-6: Moderate (from olive oil)

To meet AAFCO standards, we highly recommend adding a multivitamin to each meal. One of my favorite multivitamins that I recommend is this one.

https://amzn.to/3YpWSRI >>>

9. Pea & Sweet Potato Stew

Nutritional Information:

- » Final weight: 8 oz (230g)
- » Calories: 150 kcal
- » Proteins: 6%
- » Fats: 8%
- » Carbohydrates: 35%

Ingredients:

- » 1/2 cup (90g) cooked peas
- » 1/2 cup (90g) mashed sweet potatoes
- » 1 tsp (5ml) flaxseed oil

Instructions:

1. Cook Peas: Steam or boil peas until tender.
2. Prepare Sweet Potatoes: Boil sweet potatoes until tender, then mash.
3. Combine Ingredients: Mix peas and mashed sweet potatoes in a bowl.
4. Add Healthy Fats: Stir in flaxseed oil before serving.

Ingredient Substitution Tips:

- » Replace sweet potatoes with pumpkin for a different texture.
- » Use green beans instead of peas for a milder flavor.

Vitamins and Minerals:

- » Vitamin A: High (from sweet potatoes)
- » Fiber: Moderate (from peas)
- » Omega-3: Moderate (from flaxseed oil)

To meet AAFCO standards, we highly recommend adding a multivitamin to each meal. One of my favorite multivitamins that I recommend is this one.

https://amzn.to/3YpWSRI >>>

10. Pumpkin & Spinach Medley

Nutritional Information:

» Final weight: 8 oz (230g)

» Calories: 130 kcal

» Proteins: 6%

» Fats: 8%

» Carbohydrates: 30%

Ingredients:

» 1/2 cup (90g) cooked pumpkin (pureed)

» 1/2 cup (90g) steamed spinach

» 1 tsp (5ml) olive oil

Instructions:

1. Prepare Pumpkin: Steam or bake pumpkin, then puree it.
2. Steam Spinach: Steam spinach until wilted.
3. Combine Ingredients: Mix pumpkin and spinach in a bowl.
4. Add Healthy Fats: Stir in olive oil before serving.

Ingredient Substitution Tips:

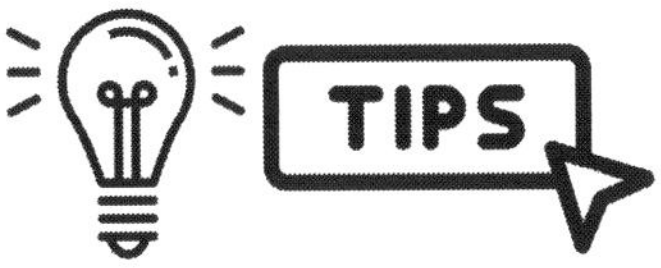

» Replace pumpkin with sweet potatoes for a more substantial dish.

» Use kale instead of spinach for more texture.

Vitamins and Minerals:

» Vitamin A: High (from pumpkin)

» Iron: High (from spinach)

» Omega-6: Moderate (from olive oil)

To meet AAFCO standards, we highly recommend adding a multivitamin to each meal. One of my favorite multivitamins that I recommend is this one.

https://amzn.to/3YpWSRI >>>

CHAPTER 4: ADDRESSING DIETARY RESTRICTIONS & HEALTH CONCERNS

Making meals for dogs with dietary restrictions or health issues requires careful thought and attention to their needs. Preparing homemade meals ensures your dog gets the right nutrition, tailored to avoid allergens and harmful ingredients. This is especially important for dogs with allergies, or other health concerns. Knowing exactly what goes into your dog's food gives you peace of mind.

Let's take a look at how to identify common food allergies and manage them through diet. We'll also cover how to run elimination diets to find specific allergens, along with tips to prevent cross-contamination in homes with multiple pets.

IDENTIFYING COMMON FOOD ALLERGIES

Wheat

Wheat is often used in dog food as a filler. This means it is included to bulk up the food without providing much nutritional value. While not every dog is allergic to wheat, it can lead to problems for those who are sensitive. Symptoms of a wheat allergy can include skin irritation and persistent itching. Some dogs may experience digestive issues, such as diarrhea or vomiting, after consuming wheat as well.

If you suspect that your dog might have a wheat allergy, consider switching to grain-free options. There are many alternative foods available that do not contain wheat or other grains. Look for brands that use ingredients like sweet potatoes or brown rice instead. These options can provide necessary carbohydrates without the risks associated with wheat.

Chicken

Chicken is another ingredient commonly found in dog food. It is often praised for being a good source of protein, which is essential for a dog's growth and energy. However, just like with wheat, some dogs can develop an allergy to chicken. Signs of a chicken allergy may include ear infections, itching, or even upset stomach.

In cases where a chicken allergy is suspected, it's important to switch to a different protein source. There are many meat alternatives that can be as nutritious. For example, consider feeding your dog turkey, lamb, or fish. These meats can provide high-quality protein without the risk of allergic reactions, making them suitable substitutes.

Beef

Beef is another common allergen found in commercial dog foods. Many dog food brands include beef as a primary protein source because it is appealing to dogs and often more affordable. However, beef allergies can manifest as symptoms like itching, skin infections, and gastrointestinal issues.

For dog owners noticing signs of a beef allergy, identifying an appropriate alternative is necessary. A good approach would be to switch to a diet that features novel proteins. That could include ingredients like bison or venison. These meats are less likely to have been previously consumed, thereby decreasing the chance of allergic reactions.

Recognizing Allergy Symptoms

It's important to spot food allergies early. Signs include itching, scratching, licking, or chewing paws, ears, or skin. Digestive issues like vomiting, diarrhea, or gas are also common. Sometimes, allergies show up as changes in energy levels, weight, or even behavior. Catching these signs early allows you to make changes before the problem worsens.

Using an Elimination Diet

One way to find out if your dog has a food allergy is through an elimination diet. This means feeding your dog a special diet with no ingredients they've eaten before, for 8-12 weeks. During this time, avoid giving any other foods, treats, or supplements to prevent cross-contamination. If your dog's symptoms improve, you can reintroduce the old food to see if the allergy returns. If it does, you'll know that food is the cause.

Running an elimination diet takes planning. Clean all food bowls thoroughly and stick strictly to the new diet. You can mix the new food with their regular food over a few days to prevent stomach upset. Prescription diets are often recommended because they meet the necessary standards. In some cases, homemade diets using safe proteins may be needed.

Working with a Veterinarian

It's important to work with your vet throughout this process. They can help you choose the right diet and make sure it's balanced. Vets can also run tests to confirm allergies and suggest supplements if needed. Veterinary dermatologists specialize in diagnosing and managing food allergies, making them a great resource for advice.

Avoiding Cross-Contamination

If you have more than one pet, make sure they eat separately during feeding times to avoid contamination. Clean up bowls right after feeding, and consider putting all pets on the same diet to make things easier. Slowly introducing a new diet helps avoid additional digestive problems.

Tracking Symptoms

During the elimination diet, keep a journal of any changes in your dog's symptoms. Reintroduce old foods one at a time to figure out which ingredient is causing the allergic reaction. This careful approach ensures you get clear results.

Creating a Long-Term Diet

Once you know which foods to avoid, you and your vet can create a long-term diet. There are many hypoallergenic options available, both commercial and homemade. If you choose to cook at home, make sure to include any necessary supplements to keep your dog's diet balanced.

CREATING LOW-FAT MEALS FOR WEIGHT MANAGEMENT

Maintaining a healthy weight in dogs is crucial for preventing obesity-related issues like diabetes, arthritis, and heart disease. Excess weight can strain a dog's joints and organs, reducing their quality of life and longevity. Preparing low-fat meals at home, tailored to your dog's needs, is a proactive step in supporting their long-term health.

Low-Fat Recipe 1: Lean Turkey and Pumpkin Dish

A lean turkey and pumpkin dish is a simple, nutritious meal that helps manage your dog's weight. This recipe combines lean turkey, rich in protein and low in fat, with pumpkin, which is great for digestion due to its fiber content.

Ingredients:

» 500 grams (1 lb) of lean ground turkey

» 1 cup of cooked, mashed pumpkin

» 1/2 cup of chopped carrots (optional)

» 1/2 cup of green beans (optional)

» 1 tablespoon of fish oil (for omega-3 fatty acids)

Nutritional Information (per serving, approx. 1 cup):

» Calories: 250

» Protein: 27g

» Fat: 8g

» Carbohydrates: 14g

» Fiber: 5g

Instructions:

1. Cook Beef: Sauté lean ground beef until cooked through, drain any excess fat.
2. Prepare Rice: Cook brown rice according to package instructions.
3. Steam Carrots: Steam or boil carrots until tender, dice into small pieces.
4. Combine Ingredients: Mix beef, rice, and carrots together.
5. Add Healthy Fats: Stir in olive oil and serve once cooled.

Vitamins and Minerals:

» Omega-3 Fatty Acids: High (due to fish oil)

» Vitamins/Minerals: High in vitamins A, C, and potassium (from pumpkin)

This meal is low in fat yet full of vitamins, minerals, and fiber. The added vegetables provide extra nutrients while keeping the calorie count low. Properly cooking the ingredients makes the food easier to digest and more enjoyable for your dog.

To meet AAFCO standards, we highly recommend adding a multivitamin to each meal. One of my favorite multivitamins that I recommend is this one.

https://amzn.to/3YpWSRI >>>

Low-Fat Recipe 2: Hearty Vegetable Stew

This hearty vegetable stew is packed with low-calorie, nutrient-dense ingredients to help your dog feel full without the extra calories.

Ingredients:

- » 1 cup of chopped sweet potatoes
- » 1 cup of chopped zucchini
- » 1 cup of chopped spinach
- » 1/2 cup of green peas
- » 2 tablespoons of olive oil
- » 4 cups of water or low-sodium chicken broth

Nutritional Information (per serving, approx. 1 cup):

- » Calories: 190
- » Protein: 5g
- » Fat: 9g
- » Carbohydrates: 22g
- » Fiber: 6g

Instructions:

1. In a large pot, combine the sweet potatoes, zucchini, spinach, and peas.
2. Add the water or chicken broth and bring to a boil.
3. Reduce the heat and let it simmer until all the vegetables are tender.
4. Stir in the olive oil.
5. Allow the stew to cool before serving.

Vitamins and Minerals:

- » High in vitamins A, C, K, and potassium (from vegetables), good source of iron and calcium

This stew is rich in vitamins A, C, and K, along with iron and calcium, thanks to the variety of vegetables. The low-sodium chicken broth adds flavor without extra salt or calories, making this meal a healthy, flavorful option.

To meet AAFCO standards, we highly recommend adding a multivitamin to each meal. One of my favorite multivitamins that I recommend is this one.

https://amzn.to/3YpWSRl >>>

Practical Portion Control Tips

Portion control is essential for managing your dog's weight. Here are some practical tips to prevent overfeeding:

Measure Portions: Use a kitchen scale or measuring cups to accurately portion your dog's food. Guessing can easily lead to overfeeding. Check out Vet Approved for our recommendations 137.

Create a Feeding Schedule: Stick to regular meal times each day to avoid hunger between meals, which can lead to begging or scavenging.

Monitor Body Condition: Regularly assess your dog's weight and body condition, and adjust their portions as needed.

Avoid Table Scraps: As tempting as it can be, avoid giving your dog food from the table so they can stick to their diet that you have made.

Use Smaller Bowls: Serve meals in smaller bowls to make portions appear larger, helping your dog feel more satisfied.

FORMULATING MEALS FOR DIABETIC DOGS

Canine diabetes occurs when the pancreas doesn't produce enough insulin or when the body's cells become resistant to insulin. This leads to high blood sugar levels, resulting in symptoms like increased thirst, frequent urination, and weight loss. Proper dietary management, combined with insulin therapy, is key to stabilizing blood sugar levels.

Insulin helps glucose enter the body's cells to be used for energy. Without enough insulin, glucose stays in the bloodstream, causing high blood sugar. Administering insulin as prescribed by a vet and timing meals correctly is crucial. Feeding your dog at regular intervals (typically every 10-12 hours) helps maintain steady blood sugar levels, reducing the risk of hypoglycemia (low blood sugar) or hyperglycemia (high blood sugar).

Recipe 1: Chicken & Quinoa Meal for Diabetic Dogs

This protein-rich, low-glycemic meal helps stabilize blood sugar while providing essential nutrients for your diabetic dog.

Nutritional Information (per serving, approx. 1 cup):

- » Calories: 290
- » Protein: 30g
- » Fat: 10g
- » Carbohydrates: 18g
- » Fiber: 4g

Ingredients:

- » 1 cup cooked, shredded skinless chicken breast
- » 1/2 cup cooked quinoa
- » 1/4 cup steamed broccoli florets (chopped)
- » 1/4 cup steamed carrots (diced)
- » 1 tablespoon flaxseed oil

Instructions:

1. Cook the chicken breast thoroughly and shred it into small pieces.
2. Prepare the quinoa according to the package instructions, then let it cool.
3. Steam the broccoli and carrots until tender, then chop into small pieces.
4. Combine all ingredients in a large bowl and mix well.
5. Add the flaxseed oil and stir to evenly distribute.

Vitamins and Minerals:

- » Omega-3 Fatty Acids: High (due to flaxseed oil)
- » Vitamins/Minerals: High in vitamins A, C, and potassium (from vegetables)

This meal is rich in high-quality protein from the chicken, essential for muscle maintenance, and includes quinoa, a low-glycemic grain that prevents rapid blood sugar spikes. The added vegetables provide vitamins and minerals, while flaxseed oil adds healthy fats.

To meet AAFCO standards, we highly recommend adding a multivitamin to each meal. One of my favorite multivitamins that I recommend is this one.

https://amzn.to/3YpWSRI >>>

Recipe 2: Grain-Free Fish & Vegetable Dish

This grain-free recipe promotes better blood sugar control and provides healthy fats and fiber to support overall health.

Nutritional Information (per serving, approx. 1 cup):

- Calories: 260
- Protein: 25g
- Fat: 12g
- Carbohydrates: 15g
- Fiber: 5g

Ingredients:

- 1 cup cooked, flaked salmon
- 1/2 cup roasted sweet potatoes (diced)
- 1/4 cup steamed green beans (chopped)
- 1/4 cup lightly wilted spinach
- 1 tablespoon olive oil

Instructions:

1. Cook the salmon and flake it into small pieces, removing any bones.
2. Roast the sweet potatoes until soft, then dice into small cubes.
3. Steam the green beans and chop them into bite-sized pieces.
4. Lightly wilt the spinach in a pan over low heat.
5. Combine all ingredients in a large bowl and mix thoroughly.
6. Drizzle with olive oil and stir to coat.

Vitamins and Minerals:

- Omega-3 Fatty Acids: High (due to salmon and olive oil)
- Vitamins/Minerals: High in vitamins A, C, K, and fiber (from vegetables)

Salmon provides omega-3 fatty acids, which support heart health and have anti-inflammatory properties. Sweet potatoes, a low-glycemic option, regulate blood sugar, while green beans and spinach offer essential nutrients and antioxidants. Olive oil adds healthy fats, supporting your dog's overall well-being.

To meet AAFCO standards, we highly recommend adding a multivitamin to each meal. One of my favorite multivitamins that I recommend is this one... https://amzn.to/3YpWSRl

Monitoring Your Diabetic Dog's Health

It's important to monitor how your dog responds to these homemade meals. Regular blood sugar checks using a glucometer provide valuable insights into how well their diet and insulin therapy are working. Keep a consistent log of blood glucose levels and share them with your vet during checkups.

Frequent weigh-ins are also recommended, especially if your dog is overweight or underweight. Maintaining an ideal weight plays a significant role in managing diabetes. Overweight dogs may need a diet higher in fiber to promote fullness without extra calories, while underweight dogs might require additional protein and fat to help them reach a healthy weight.

Crafting homemade meals for dogs with dietary restrictions doesn't have to be challenging. Always remember to consult with a veterinarian to ensure nutritional balance and monitor your dog's response to new diets.

CHAPTER 5: STRUCTURED MEAL PLANS FOR DOGS

Creating structured meal plans can greatly improve your dog's overall health and well-being. With a well-organized plan, you can meet your dog's specific nutritional needs, whether you have a French Bulldog or a large Labrador. Structured meal plans offer numerous benefits, including preventing health issues and ensuring your dog gets the right balance of nutrients every day.

You'll learn how to develop meal plans tailored to your dog's size, activity level, and lifestyle. We'll cover key topics such as determining caloric intake based on activity, including nutrient-dense organ meats, and balancing them with other food types. You'll also find guidance on monitoring your dog's weight and adjusting portions to avoid overfeeding or underfeeding. For dogs with allergies or sensitivities, we'll provide tips on making gradual dietary changes and offer a 30-day meal plan to simplify the transition to homemade meals. Whether your dog is highly active or prefers lounging around, the information here will help you create a diet plan that supports their long-term health.

30-DAY MEAL PLAN FOR DOGS: A MONTHLY GUIDE

Implementing a structured meal plan requires paying attention to your dog's specific nutritional needs, especially for large breeds that are prone to joint and bone issues. A diet that supports joint health is essential. As a vet, the one thing I always tell my patients is to consider adding supplements like glucosamine to maintain healthy cartilage and joints. DHA and omega-6 fatty acids also support joint health. Starting these supplements early can significantly benefit your dog's long-term joint health. For a list of vet approved supplements check out my Vet Approved on page 140.

Here's a sample meal plan to guide you through a full month of tailored meals. Remember, this is just an example, and adjustments may be necessary based on your dog's specific needs:

Week 1

» Day 1: Beef & Brown Rice Bowl

» Day 2: Sweet Potato & Pea Mash (Vegetable-Based)

» Day 3: Venison & Sweet Potato Hash

» Day 4: Turkey & Quinoa Breakfast Bowl

» Day 5: Salmon & Sweet Potato Mash

» Day 6: Carrot & Zucchini Blend (Vegetable-Based)

» Day 7: Chicken & Barley Stew

Week 2

» Day 8: Pork & Barley Stew

» Day 9: Spinach & Sweet Potato Medley (Vegetable-Based)

» Day 10: Ground Beef & Sweet Potato Mix

- Day 11: Turkey & Barley Stew
- Day 12: Cod & Carrot Blend
- Day 13: Lamb & Carrot Stew
- Day 14: Pumpkin & Carrot Bowl (Vegetable-Based)

Week 3

- Day 15: Beef Heart & Rice Mix
- Day 16: Chicken & Green Bean Blend
- Day 17: Turkey & Sweet Potato Hash
- Day 18: Tuna & Barley Stew
- Day 19: Green Bean & Sweet Potato Mash (Vegetable-Based)
- Day 20: Pork Liver & Barley Stew
- Day 21: Chicken & Spinach Stew

Week 4

- Day 22: Beef Liver & Pumpkin Mix
- Day 23: Kale & Carrot Blend (Vegetable-Based)
- Day 24: Turkey & Zucchini Stew
- Day 25: Sardine & Quinoa Mix
- Day 26: Ground Beef & Zucchini Medley
- Day 27: Chicken & Pumpkin Bowl
- Day 28: Mackerel & Brown Rice Mix
- Day 29: Broccoli & Pumpkin Mix (Vegetable-Based)
- Day 30: Cod & Green Bean Medley

Guideline: Record any noticeable changes in your dog's behavior or health.

Throughout the month, remember to stick to the structured plan but remain flexible in case of any adverse reactions. Keep an eye on your dog's energy levels, coat condition, and overall demeanor, as these can be indicators of how well the diet is working. The goal is to maintain a balanced approach, providing all necessary nutrients without causing stress to your dog's digestive system.

CUSTOMIZED MEAL PLANS BASED ON ACTIVITY LEVEL

When designing meal plans for dogs, it's important to consider their individual activity levels. Dogs' energy needs vary greatly depending on factors like age and breed, so meal plans must be tailored accordingly to ensure they stay healthy and have enough energy.

Activity Levels: Low, Moderate, and High

1. Low activity dogs: These include older dogs or those with sedentary lifestyles. They need fewer calories but still require balanced nutrition to maintain health. For example, a senior Chihuahua will have different caloric needs than a younger, more active terrier.

2. Moderate activity dogs: These dogs engage in regular exercise, like daily walks or play sessions. Breeds like Beagles or Cocker Spaniels often fall into this category.

3. High activity dogs: These dogs participate in intense physical activities, such as agility training, herding, or long-distance running. Breeds like Border Collies and German Shepherds are prime examples.

Age and Breed Influence Energy Needs

Puppies need more calories per pound than adult dogs because they grow quickly and have higher energy levels.

Senior dogs slow down with age and usually require fewer calories.

Working breeds, like Huskies, generally have higher energy needs than smaller, toy breeds like Pomeranians.

Nutritional Needs for Active Dogs

For dogs with higher activity levels, a protein-rich diet is crucial. Proteins support muscle recovery and overall growth, helping maintain body tissues. Animal proteins like chicken, beef, and fish provide essential amino acids that dogs can't produce on their own.

Carbohydrates also play a key role in providing sustained energy. Complex carbs like sweet potatoes and brown rice release energy slowly, helping dogs maintain consistent activity levels throughout the day.

Hydration for Active Dogs

Dehydration is a common concern for highly active dogs. Signs of dehydration include excessive panting, dry gums, lethargy, and sunken eyes. To prevent dehydration, consider adding water-rich foods to their diet, like cucumbers, watermelon, and low-sodium broths. Fresh water should always be available.

Seasonal Changes and Nutritional Needs

Dogs' nutritional needs can change with the seasons. In colder months, they may need more calories to maintain their body temperature, while in warmer months, they might eat less but require more hydration. Gradually adjusting meal plans during these times helps prevent sudden weight changes. Monitoring your dog's weight closely during seasonal transitions ensures they receive the right balance of nutrients.

ADJUSTING MEAL PLANS OVER TIME

Flexibility in meal planning is key to keeping your dog's diet balanced and meeting their changing needs. It's important to recognize signs of health issues early, such as changes in weight. Regular weigh-ins and monitoring your dog's body condition can help you spot underlying problems. For example, sudden weight loss could point to digestive issues or metabolic disorders, while rapid weight gain might indicate hypothyroidism or overfeeding.

Always consult your veterinarian when you notice weight changes. They can provide tailored advice and make sure any dietary adjustments are suitable for your dog's health. Working with a vet also helps prevent drastic changes that could cause stress or nutrient imbalances. Vets can also run tests to pinpoint the cause of the weight change, allowing for precise adjustments to the diet.

Adapting Diets for Senior Dogs

As dogs age, their nutritional needs shift. Senior dogs generally need fewer calories because of decreased activity, but their meals should remain nutritionally rich. Lowering calorie intake while increasing fiber can help with weight management and digestion. Fiber-rich foods also help prevent constipation, a common issue in older dogs. Adding vegetables and whole grains ensures your dog gets the right vitamins and minerals without unnecessary calories.

It's also helpful to add joint supplements like glucosamine and chondroitin to support joint health. Omega-3 fatty acids, found in fish oil, reduce inflammation and maintain skin and coat health. This balanced approach helps keep senior dogs active, preventing weight gain and nutritional deficiencies.

Managing Weight Issues

For overweight dogs, high-protein diets combined with low-GI (glycemic index) ingredients, like carrots, broccoli, and butternut squash, can provide steady energy without spiking blood sugar. This helps reduce the risk of diabetes and supports gradual weight loss. Underweight dogs, on the other hand, may need more calorie-dense foods like lamb or beef. Ensuring the food is easily digestible helps maintain muscle mass and overall health.

Adding anti-inflammatory ingredients like blueberries or green tea extract can help manage weight and boost your dog's metabolism and immune system. Portion control is also critical, measuring meals accurately ensures your dog gets the right amount of food to meet their energy needs. This approach helps improve muscle-to-fat ratios and overall vitality.

Seasonal Adjustments to Meal Plans

Your dog's dietary needs change with the seasons. In summer, dogs are usually more active and may need more energy. Meals rich in lean proteins and hydrating fruits like watermelon can keep them energized and hydrated. These foods offer essential nutrients and help maintain hydration in hot weather.

In winter, when dogs are less active, reducing calorie intake helps prevent weight gain. Fiber-rich vegetables and low-calorie foods, like sweet potatoes, are great choices because they provide warmth and sustenance without excess calories. It's also important to ensure consistent water intake during colder months. Adding warm broths to meals can encourage drinking and keep your dog hydrated.

Adjusting meal plans based on seasonal changes not only meets your dog's shifting energy needs but also keeps their diet varied and exciting. Dogs, like humans, benefit from variety in their meals, and seasonal adjustments ensure they receive the right balance of nutrients all year long.

MONITORING WEIGHT CHANGES

Assessing Your Dog's Weight: Weigh-Ins and Body Condition Scoring (BCS)

Regular weigh-ins and body condition scoring (BCS) are essential tools for monitoring your dog's health and ensuring they maintain a healthy weight. Weighing your dog consistently allows you to detect any fluctuations that could signal underlying health concerns. A simple routine could involve weighing your dog weekly or bi-weekly using a reliable scale, and keeping a record of the results to track trends over time.

Body condition scoring complements weigh-ins by providing a visual and hands-on method to assess your dog's physique. The BCS system typically ranges from one to nine:

1-3: Underweight, with visible ribs, spine, and no fat cover.

4-5: Ideal weight, where ribs are easily felt without excess fat, and your dog has a discernible waist.

6-9: Overweight to obese, with thick fat layers, no visible waist, and difficulty feeling the ribs.

To conduct a BCS at home, observe your dog from above and from the side. You should see a noticeable waistline from above and feel the ribs without excess fat. For dogs with thick coats, press lightly to get an accurate feel. Aim for a BCS of 4-5 for most dogs, which indicates an ideal body condition.

Adjusting Meal Portions Based on Weight and BCS

Once you determine your dog's weight and BCS, you can adjust their food portions accordingly. If your dog is gaining weight, reduce their caloric intake slightly and monitor the changes. If they are underweight, gradually increase their food portions to ensure they receive the necessary nutrients. Always use a measuring cup to portion food accurately—guesswork can easily lead to overfeeding or underfeeding.

For specific recommendations, consult your veterinarian. They can provide tailored guidance on adjusting food portions based on your dog's breed, age, and activity level.

Signs of Overfeeding and Underfeeding

Recognizing the signs of overfeeding or underfeeding is key to maintaining your dog's health:

Overfeeding can lead to rapid weight gain, lethargy, and difficulty moving due to joint strain. Overfed dogs might also have a distended belly and be at risk for conditions like diabetes, arthritis, or heart disease.

Underfeeding may result in malnutrition, a dull coat, visible ribs, and decreased energy. These symptoms indicate your dog isn't getting enough nutrients to sustain their health.

Monitoring these signs helps you make necessary adjustments before minor issues escalate into more serious health concerns.

Consistency and Flexibility in Meal Planning

Maintaining a consistent routine with your dog's meal schedule helps prevent sudden weight fluctuations and makes it easier to identify any irregularities in their health. Stick to regular feeding times and closely monitor your dog's reaction to any dietary changes. If you notice significant shifts in their appetite, energy levels, or physical appearance, review their diet and consult your vet.

Consistency is important, but so is flexibility. Be ready to adjust your dog's meal plan as needed, based on changes in their activity level, age, or health. Puppies and active adult dogs often require more calories than senior dogs or those with a sedentary lifestyle. If your dog's activity level changes due to new exercise routines or seasonal shifts, adjust their portions accordingly.

Exercise

Incorporating physical activity into your dog's routine is just as important as managing their diet. Exercise not only helps maintain a healthy weight but also improves your dog's overall well-being and mood. Aim for at least 30 minutes of activity per day, adjusting the intensity and type of exercise based on your dog's breed, age, and health. Activities like walking, running, or playing fetch can help keep your dog fit and engaged.

CHAPTER 6: TOOLS AND RESOURCES FOR SUCCESS

In this chapter, we'll cover essential tools and resources for successful homemade dog meal preparation. You'll learn about conversion tables to help with ingredient measurements, ensuring precise nutrient balances. We'll also discuss serving size charts tailored to different breeds and weights to make sure you're feeding the correct portions. In addition, we'll provide nutritional breakdowns of common ingredients so you can make informed choices when planning meals. This comprehensive guide equips you with everything needed to transition seamlessly to nutritious, homemade dog food.

CONVERSION TABLES FOR INGREDIENT MEASUREMENTS

Accurately measuring ingredients for homemade dog food is key to providing a nutritionally balanced diet. This section will guide you through understanding different measurement units, converting common ingredients, creating a DIY conversion chart, and tips for measuring accuracy.

Understanding Measurement Units

Dog food recipes often use both volume (e.g., cups, teaspoons, tablespoons) and weight (e.g., grams, ounces) measurements. Volume measurements are convenient for quick reference, but weight measurements are far more accurate for ensuring nutritional balance. The weight of ingredients can vary depending on their density, so a cup of one ingredient might weigh significantly more or less than a cup of another. For instance, a cup of kibble weighs differently than a cup of rice, which could affect the meal's overall nutritional content.

Common Ingredient Conversions

Knowing how to convert between volume and weight is essential for precise meal preparation. Here are conversions for some commonly used dog food ingredients:

- **Chicken breast:** 1 cup diced = approximately 140 grams
- **Brown rice:** 1 cup cooked = around 195 grams
- **Oats:** 1 cup = roughly 90 grams
- **Sweet potatoes:** 1 cup mashed = about 200 grams
- **Carrots:** 1 cup chopped = nearly 130 grams

These conversions make it easier to adjust recipes or modify portion sizes. Understanding these measurements ensures you're providing the right amount of each ingredient, contributing to a balanced diet for your dog.

Creating a Personalized Conversion Chart

Building your own conversion chart for frequently used ingredients can save time and ensure consistency in your homemade dog meals. To create a DIY conversion chart, measure out a cup or other volume of your most commonly used ingredients, then weigh them on a kitchen scale. Write down the measurements, and soon you'll have a quick-reference guide customized to your cooking habits. Keep this chart in your kitchen for easy access whenever you prepare meals.

TIPS FOR MEASURING ACCURACY

The most reliable way to measure ingredients is by using a kitchen scale. Weighing ingredients instead of relying on volume measurements reduces inaccuracies caused by differences in ingredient density. For example, dry ingredients like kibble or grains can vary in weight even if they take up the same amount of space, leading to overfeeding or underfeeding. Accurate measurements help prevent giving too many calories (which can lead to weight gain) or too few (which can cause malnutrition).

TIP - For my budget friendly scales see page 139.

Here are a few tips to ensure accuracy:

Tare your scale: Before measuring each ingredient, place your bowl or container on the scale and press the tare button to zero it out. This way, you're only measuring the ingredient itself, not the container.

Measure ingredients close to feeding time: Ingredients can lose moisture or change weight over time, especially if they've been frozen or exposed to air. Measure as close to the time of feeding as possible to ensure accurate measurements.

Use proper technique for volume measurements: When measuring dry ingredients, like flour, spoon it into the cup and level it off without packing it down. For liquids, measure at eye level to get an accurate reading. Use measuring spoons for smaller quantities like oils or supplements, and ensure they're filled to the brim and leveled off.

Consistency is key: Use the same measuring tools and methods each time to keep portions consistent and balanced. Keeping your measuring tools clean and using the same ones regularly will help maintain accuracy over time.

By following these tips, you can ensure that every meal you prepare is as nutritionally balanced as possible, helping prevent health issues related to inaccurate feeding practices.

SERVING SIZE CHARTS FOR DIFFERENT BREEDS AND WEIGHTS

To ensure your dog is getting the right portion size, it's important to refer to serving size charts based on their breed and weight. Dogs have varying caloric needs depending on their size, age, and activity level. Small breeds like Chihuahuas or Dachshunds have different energy requirements compared to larger breeds like Labradors or Great Danes.

Serving size charts, which can often be found online or provided by veterinarians, help guide you in determining the correct portion sizes. Using these charts, combined with the precise measurements from your conversion tables, ensures that you're feeding your dog appropriately for their size and lifestyle.

Dog Portion Size Chart

Dog Breed/ Weight Range	Daily Calories	Portion Size per Meal (cups)	Meals per Day	Activity Level
Small (up to 10 lbs)	200-400	0.5 - 1	2	Low to moderate
Medium (10-25 lbs)	400-600	1 - 1.5	2	Low to moderate
Large (25-50 lbs)	800-1200	1.5 - 2.5	2	Moderate to high
Extra Large (50+ lbs)	1200-2000	2.5 - 4	2	Moderate to high

In addition to static charts, modern technology offers interactive tools to help customize serving sizes for your dog's unique needs. An interactive serving size calculator is a valuable resource for pet owners. These calculators often require inputs like your dog's breed, weight, age, activity level, and sometimes even specific health issues. By entering this information, these tools provide a personalized feeding recommendation.

Using these calculators can simplify meal planning and ensure you're providing the best possible care tailored to your dog's individual requirements. Here are some to get your started:

1. **Pawtrack:** A app specifically designed for tracking feeding times, exercise, and health records with reminders for vet appointments and medication.

2. **Dog Log:** This app allows you to track your dog's training, health, and daily activities, including feeding times.

3. **Pet First Aid:** While focused on first aid, this app also provides health tracking features and feeding schedules.

4. **My Dog's Diary:** A comprehensive diary app for tracking your dog's diet, weight, and health progress.

5. **WoofTrax:** Primarily a walking app, it also helps you log feeding times and health records.

6. **PetDesk:** Helps manage vet appointments, vaccinations, and includes a feature for tracking feeding schedules.

Lastly, maintaining a feeding diary can be a useful tool for tracking what your dog eats daily. This record can highlight any patterns or changes in eating habits that might indicate health issues. It also provides a clear picture for your vet during consultations, helping them make more informed recommendations.

Accurately measuring ingredients is a critical step in ensuring your dog's homemade meals are nutritionally balanced. Remember, the goal is to provide a well-rounded diet that supports your dog's health and well-being.

CHAPTER 7: HYGIENE AND SAFETY IN HOMEMADE DOG FOOD

Maintaining proper hygiene and safety when preparing homemade dog food is crucial for your dog's overall health and well-being. As a pet owner, preparing meals at home gives you full control over the ingredients, allowing you to ensure that your dog is eating nutritious, high-quality food. However, this also comes with the responsibility of adhering to strict hygiene practices to protect your pet from harmful bacteria and contamination. Neglecting food safety can lead to foodborne illnesses that can affect both your dog and your household.

SAFE FOOD HANDLING PRACTICES

Safe food handling is the foundation of preparing healthy, homemade meals for your dog. Following these practices minimizes the risk of bacterial contamination and ensures that your dog's food remains clean and safe to eat.

1. Handwashing: The First Line of Defense

One of the most important steps in food preparation is handwashing. Proper hand hygiene prevents the spread of bacteria and other contaminants to your dog's food. According to the Centers for Disease Control and Prevention (CDC), you should scrub your hands with soap and warm water for at least 20 seconds. Pay special attention to the spaces between your fingers and under your nails, where bacteria can easily hide.

It's essential to wash your hands before you start cooking, after handling raw meat or eggs, and before touching any ready-to-eat food. This practice not only protects your dog from potential foodborne illnesses but also keeps you and your family safe from contaminants that could transfer from raw ingredients.

2. Sanitizing Tools and Surfaces

Keeping your kitchen clean is just as important as ensuring your dog's food is nutritious. Surfaces, cutting boards, and utensils can harbor bacteria if they are not properly sanitized. Before starting any meal preparation, make sure all tools, including knives, spoons, and cutting boards, are thoroughly washed and sanitized.

Use a disinfectant solution or hot, soapy water to clean countertops, cutting boards, and utensils before and after food preparation. For even better results, use a dishwasher with a sanitize cycle to clean utensils and dishes. Regularly sanitize any areas where raw meat is handled to prevent the spread of bacteria like E. coli and Salmonella.

3. Designating Food Prep Areas for Your Dog

Cross-contamination can occur when dog food preparation areas and utensils are shared with those used for human food. To prevent this, designate specific areas in your kitchen for preparing your dog's food. Ideally, this should be a separate countertop or space to avoid confusion and contamination. If space is limited, at least ensure that all surfaces are thoroughly cleaned and sanitized before switching from human food to pet food preparation.

In addition, label specific utensils, cutting boards, and containers as "dog-only" items. This can prevent the accidental use of these items for human food, further reducing the risk of contamination. In households with multiple people, it's helpful to communicate these practices to everyone to maintain consistency in food safety.

See our Vet Approved section for all our favorite utensils and items (page 139)!

PREVENTING CROSS-CONTAMINATION

Cross-contamination is one of the primary ways bacteria spread in the kitchen. Preventing it requires careful attention to how different ingredients and surfaces are handled during food preparation. Here are some key practices to prevent cross-contamination when preparing homemade dog food.

1. Separate Cutting Boards for Raw Meat and Vegetables

One of the most effective ways to prevent cross-contamination is by using separate cutting boards for raw meat and plant-based ingredients. Raw meat, poultry, and fish can contain harmful bacteria that could be transferred to vegetables or other ready-to-eat ingredients. By keeping raw and cooked ingredients separate, you reduce the risk of spreading pathogens like Salmonella, E. coli, or Campylobacter, which can cause illness in both dogs and humans.

Choose color-coded cutting boards to easily distinguish between boards used for meat and those for other ingredients. Clean and sanitize each board after use to ensure that no bacteria are left behind.

2. Proper Storage of Ingredients and Prepared Meals

Storing ingredients and prepared meals correctly is essential for preventing bacterial growth. Raw meat should always be kept in sealed containers and stored separately from other foods in your refrigerator or freezer. Place raw meat on the bottom shelf of your refrigerator to prevent juices from dripping onto other foods.

When you've prepared a batch of homemade dog food, use airtight containers to store it in the fridge or freezer. This prevents the food from being exposed to air and moisture, which can cause spoilage and bacterial growth. Be sure to label containers with the date and the type of food so you can use the oldest batches first, reducing food waste and keeping meals fresh.

3. Cleaning as You Go

Cleaning up spills and messes as soon as they happen is an important part of maintaining a hygienic kitchen. Bacteria can quickly spread on countertops and utensils, so it's crucial to wipe down surfaces regularly with hot, soapy water or a disinfectant. Keeping your kitchen tidy as you prepare food also minimizes the chances of contamination from dirty tools or surfaces.

INVOLVING THE HOUSEHOLD IN FOOD SAFETY

For households with multiple members, it's important to involve everyone in maintaining food safety practices. Regularly educating family members about the importance of hygiene when preparing dog food helps create a culture of cleanliness. Assigning specific tasks, such as cutting vegetables or handling raw meat, ensures that each person understands their role and follows proper protocols. This collaborative approach ensures a safer cooking environment for both people and pets.

Involving children in the process can also be a fun and educational way to teach them about food safety. Simple tasks, such as washing hands or helping to label containers, help instill good hygiene habits from an early age.

PROPER STORAGE TECHNIQUES FOR HOMEMADE DOG FOOD

Storing homemade dog food correctly is essential to maintaining its freshness, nutritional value, and safety. Unlike commercial dog food, which often contains preservatives, homemade dog food is more prone to spoilage. Proper storage techniques are therefore critical to ensuring your dog receives healthy meals without the risk of bacterial contamination.

1. Refrigeration and Freezing

After preparing a batch of homemade dog food, it's important to allow the food to cool completely before storing it. Refrigerating food while it's still warm can create an ideal environment for bacteria to grow. Once the food has cooled, it can be stored in the refrigerator for up to three days.

For those who prefer to prepare larger batches, freezing is an excellent option. Divide the food into meal-sized portions and store it in airtight containers or resealable plastic bags. Label each portion with the preparation date to ensure you use the oldest portions first. Frozen dog food can typically be stored for up to three months, but always check for freezer burn or changes in texture before feeding it to your pet.

2. Airtight Containers

Using airtight containers is essential for keeping homemade dog food fresh. These containers prevent air and moisture from getting into the food, which can lead to spoilage. Choose containers made of food-safe, non-toxic materials, such as BPA-free plastic or glass. Airtight containers also help prevent the food from absorbing odors from other items in the refrigerator.

Properly sealed containers also prevent the food from being exposed to bacteria or pests, reducing the risk of contamination.

3. Monitoring Storage Temperatures

To keep homemade dog food safe, it's essential to store it at the correct temperature. Refrigerators should be set to 40°F (4°C) or lower, and freezers should be kept at 0°F (-18°C) or lower. These temperatures slow the growth of bacteria, ensuring the food remains safe for longer.

Additionally, be mindful of how long food is left out at room temperature. Homemade dog food should not be left out for more than two hours, as bacteria can multiply rapidly in warm environments.

DETECTING SPOILED FOOD

Even with proper storage techniques, homemade dog food can sometimes go bad. It's important to know the signs of spoiled food to prevent feeding it to your dog. Changes in color, texture, or smell are strong indicators that food may have spoiled. If the food has developed a sour smell, is discolored, or has a slimy texture, discard it immediately. Feeding spoiled food can lead to digestive issues and, in severe cases, food poisoning.

By following these guidelines, you can ensure that the homemade meals you prepare for your dog remain safe, nutritious, and fresh. Proper storage and handling not only maintain the quality of the food but also protect your dog's health and well-being.

With these detailed practices in place, maintaining hygiene and safety when preparing homemade dog food becomes a natural part of your routine. These methods, though requiring some initial adjustments, will significantly enhance the safety of your kitchen and ensure that the meals you prepare for your dog are healthy, safe, and enjoyable.

CONCLUSION

As we wrap up, I want to leave you with something important: the journey you've started here doesn't end with this book. The path toward nourishing your dog with homemade meals is ongoing, filled with opportunities to explore, experiment, and learn more about what makes your dog thrive. You've taken a huge step in prioritizing their health, and that's something to be proud of.

The beauty of homemade dog food is that it's flexible and adaptable. No two dogs are the same, and as your dog grows and changes, so too can their diet. You've already gained a solid understanding of how fresh, balanced meals can transform your dog's well-being, but don't stop here. Keep exploring new ingredients, testing out different recipes, and adjusting meals to suit your dog's evolving needs. Trust yourself and trust the process.

There's always more to learn. Nutrition science is ever-evolving, and there are countless ways to tweak and improve your dog's diet as you discover more about their unique preferences and health requirements. Don't be afraid to try new things, mix up ingredients, or consult your vet about what might work best as your dog ages or faces different challenges. This isn't about perfection; it's about being mindful and intentional with every meal you prepare.

Remember, the kitchen is a place of discovery. Just as you learn new techniques or find favorite recipes, your dog benefits from variety and the thoughtful adjustments you make along the way. So keep asking questions, keep experimenting, and continue to deepen your understanding of what fuels your dog's happiness and health.

Most importantly, enjoy the process. There's something incredibly rewarding about knowing that the care and effort you put into each meal is helping your dog live their best, most vibrant life. You're not just feeding them—you're actively contributing to their quality of life, one meal at a time.

So here's to the journey ahead—one filled with creativity, learning, and, most of all, a deeper bond with your furry companion. Keep cooking, keep caring, and never stop learning. You've already made a huge difference in your dog's life, and the best part is, the adventure is just beginning.

VET APPROVED

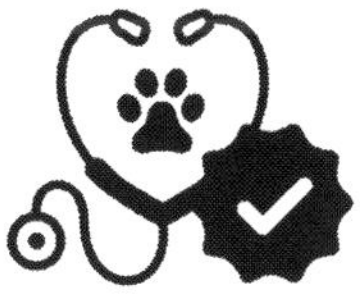

When it comes to your dog's health, you want the best—and that's why every supplement and ingredient listed here has been carefully selected and vet-approved. These products are backed by science and tailored to address your dog's specific needs, from joint support to digestive health. Incorporating these into your dog's diet can make a significant difference, enhancing their vitality, longevity, and overall well-being. Trust in these recommendations to give your dog the boost they deserve, and watch them thrive like never before. Each one of these products I have used with my own dogs and recommend to our participants at my current clinic.

» Digital Pet Scale - https://amzn.to/3MYHRAE

» Tongs - https://amzn.to/4edED8s

» Food Storage Containers - https://amzn.to/3Zxn8LN

» Food Storage Freezer Bags - https://amzn.to/3Bq2Zgq

» Plastic Cutting Board - https://amzn.to/4dhjBnZ

» Heart Dog Premium Oak Cutting Board - https://amzn.to/4gCBu3l

» Chef Knife with Self-Sharpening Blade - https://amzn.to/4eyGsfV

» Stainless Steel Measuring Cups - https://amzn.to/3ZDrEZ8

» Mixing Bowl - https://amzn.to/3TFNB6b

» Food Processor & Vegetable Chopper - https://amzn.to/3ZzUklK

» Slow Cooker - https://amzn.to/4elpFxi

» Meat Grinder - https://amzn.to/3N4k6qF

» Spatula Set - https://amzn.to/3zyN2Ei

» Non-Stick Cookware - https://amzn.to/4dnykOa

» Nonstick Carbon Steel Baking Sheet - https://amzn.to/3Ba7awP

» Vegetable Steamer Basket - https://amzn.to/3MWe37B

Supplements

» Pet Naturals Daily Multivitamin for Dogs - https://amzn.to/3YpWSRI

» Joint Health Supplement - https://amzn.to/47MG6A1

» Zesty Paws Multivitamin Treats for Dogs - https://amzn.to/4em2piC

» Purina Pro Plan Veterinary Diets FortiFlora Powder Digestive Supplement - https://amzn.to/4egzPz0

» VetriScience Composure Calming Chews for Dogs - https://amzn.to/4gLhUlw

» Zesty Paws Multivitamin Treats for Senior Dogs - https://amzn.to/4gFT4nl

» Pure Wild Alaskan Salmon Oil for Dogs - https://amzn.to/3BnFfty

» VetriScience Perio Dental Powder Dog Teeth Cleaning and Breath Freshener - https://amzn.to/3ZDhrMk

» Daily Omega-3 Supplement For Dogs - https://amzn.to/3TMN5Db

REFERENCES

A Consumer's Guide: Ensuring the Safety of Pet Food. (2021). Vt.edu. https://www.pubs.ext.vt.edu/content/pubs_ext_vt_edu/en/FST/fst-433/fst-433.html

Admin. (2019, July 24). 5 Reasons Why Your Dog May Be Losing Weight. Southseattlevet.com. https://www.southseattlevet.com/5-reasons-why-your-dog-may-be-losing-weight

American Animal Hospital Association. (2024). 5 ways to know how much to feed your pet. Retrieved from https://www.aaha.org/resources/5-ways-to-know-how-much-to-feed-your-pet/

Athena Angela Gaffud. (2024). Senior Dogs: Health Issues, Signs of Decline and What to Do. Honest Paws; Honest Paws. https://www.honestpaws.com/blogs/health/dog-senior?srsltid=AfmBOooXnoh2pmfHzHUcUgfygl3BBevkAoJEy4UqLHoikDbdUnhvG_rM

Boldan, M. (2023, June 6). Food Allergies in Dogs. Www.petmd.com. https://www.petmd.com/dog/conditions/digestive/food-allergies-dogs

Butler, M. (2023, October 31). Dog Life Stages Nutrition Guide. Nature's Logic. https://natureslogic.com/blog/dog-life-stages-nutrition-guide/

Carbo-Johnson, K. (2024). Dog vitamins & supplements: What do dogs need? Retrieved from https://www.purina.com/articles/dog/health/nutrition/types-of-supplements-for-dogs

Cline, M. G. (2024, May 2). 3 Ways Supplements Can Improve Your Dog's Joints, Digestion, and Health. Petmd.com; PetMD. https://www.petmd.com/dog/nutrition/ways-supplements-improve-dogs-joints-digestion-health

Coates, J. (2020, May 5). Are You Feeding Your Dog the Right Amount? Www.petmd.com. https://www.petmd.com/dog/nutrition/are-you-feeding-your-dog-right-amount

Common Signs of a Food Allergy in Pets | Anicira. (n.d.). Anicira.org. https://anicira.org/resources/common-signs-of-a-food-allergy-in-pets/

Cornell University College of Veterinary Medicine. (2021, July 8). Diets for diabetic dogs. https://www.vet.cornell.edu/departments-centers-and-institutes/riney-canine-health-center/canine-health-information/diets-diabetic-dogs

Diabetic Dog Diet. (2024). Vin.com. https://veterinarypartner.vin.com/doc/?id=4952921

Dog Feeding Chart: How Much Should I Feed My Dog? (n.d.). Www.purina.com. https://www.purina.com/articles/dog/feeding/guides/how-much-should-i-feed-my-dog

DVM, J. C. (2023, June 29). How to Make Vet-Approved Homemade Dog Food | Healthy Paws Pet Insurance. Pet Care Blog – Dog and Cat Health Advice and More | Healthy Paws. https://blog.healthypawspetinsurance.com/make-vet-approved-homemade-dog-food

Feb 04, J. R., Feb 04, 2019 | 7 M., & Minutes, 2019 | 7. (n.d.). How to Read a Dog Food Label. American Kennel Club. https://www.akc.org/expert-advice/nutrition/how-to-read-a-dog-food-label/

Holistic Vet Blend. (2024). Homemade dog food for skin allergies expert guide. Holistic Vet Blend. https://holisticvetblend.com/blogs/news/homemade-dog-food-for-skin-allergies-expert-guide?srsltid=AfmBOooEVW5g6fgbC6EtsXXkB5VMJKIoUt6ozkWv-hYsnalQuwvOEOop

Hospital, U. L. V. (2018, November 20). A Beginner's Guide to Home Cooking for Dogs. Union Lake Veterinary Hospital. https://unionlakeveterinaryhospital.com/blog/a-beginners-guide-to-home-cooking-for-dogs

How. (2019). How to accurately measure your pet's food. Feedingravendoodles.com. https://www.feedingravendoodles.com/articles/how-to-accurately-measure-your-pets-food

Jacobson, M. (2023, July 25). How Much Homemade Food Should I Feed? - DogCancer.com. DogCancer.com. https://www.dogcancer.com/perspectives/diet-and-lifestyle/how-much-homemade-food/

Kazimierska, K., Biel, W., Witkowicz, R., Karakulska, J., & Stachurska, X. (2021, April 26). Evaluation of nutritional value and microbiological safety in commercial dog food. Veterinary Research Communications. https://doi.org/10.1007/s11259-021-09791-6

Llera, R., & Yuill, C. (2009). Nutrition - General Feeding Guidelines for Dogs. Vca_corporate. https://vcahospitals.com/know-your-pet/nutrition-general-feeding-guidelines-for-dogs

Llera, R., Barnette, C., & Ward, E. (n.d.). Food Allergies in Dogs. Vca_corporate. https://vcahospitals.com/know-your-pet/food-allergies-in-dogs

MedVet Digital. (2024, March 12). Food Allergies in Dogs: Does My Dog Have Food Allergies? MedVet. https://www.medvet.com/food-allergy-dog/

Middleton, J. (2023, May 26). Dog food storage: All you need to know. James & Ella. https://ella.co/blog/dog-food-storage

Oct 31, M. K., Oct 31, 2019 I 4 M., & Minutes, 2019 I 4. (n.d.). Cooking For Your Dog: Pros and Cons Of Cooking Homemade Dog Food. American Kennel Club. https://www.akc.org/expert-advice/nutrition/cooking-for-your-dog-dos-and-donts/

petMD. (2011, August 4). What's in a Balanced Dog Food? I petMD. Petmd.com. https://www.petmd.com/dog/nutrition/evr_dg_whats_in_a_balanced_dog_food

philosophy. (2023, January 17). Product Handling Safety - AAFCO. AAFCO. https://www.aafco.org/resources/startups/product-handling-safety/

Raw Feeding Food Safety 101, Raw Feeding Guidance. (2019, January 11). Perfectly Rawsome. https://perfectlyrawsome.com/raw-feeding-knowledgebase/raw-feeding-food-safety-101/

Reading Labels. (n.d.). AAFCO. https://www.aafco.org/consumers/understanding-pet-food/reading-labels/

Rosling, E. (2022, June 15). Dog Nutrition Chart, Feeding & Diet Guide. Barc London; Barc London. https://www.barclondon.com/blogs/guides/dog-nutrition-chart-feeding-guide?srsltid=AfmBOopFEtjnk7Etxx3gjnNg_3E9Zn00OMssvE0wgB_xQroQypw_-a0r

Storage Safety: How to Store Dog Food - The Dog Blog I Expert Advice for Pet Parents. (2023). Bil-Jac. https://www.bil-jac.com/the-dog-blog/posts/storage-safety-how-to-store-dog-food/

Straus, M. (2008, November 12). Healthy Low-Fat Diets For Dogs With Special Dietary Needs. Whole Dog Journal. https://www.whole-dog-journal.com/health/weight_control/healthy-low-fat-diets-for-dogs-with-special-dietary-needs/

The Truth About Dog Food—an Exposé Every Dog Lover Needs to Read. (2015, July 2). The Dog People by Rover.com. https://www.rover.com/blog/dog-food-expose/

Tupler, T. (2020, September 15). How to Keep Giant Dog Breeds Healthy at Every Life Stage. Petmd.com; PetMD. https://www.petmd.com/dog/general-health/how-keep-giant-dog-breeds-healthy-every-life-stage

Vecchiato, C. G., Schwaiger, K., Biagi, G., & Dobenecker, B. (2022, September 13). From Nutritional Adequacy to Hygiene Quality: A Detailed Assessment of Commercial Raw Pet-Food for Dogs and Cats. Animals. https://doi.org/10.3390/ani12182395.

Printed in Great Britain
by Amazon

0eb1a096-5fc5-40f4-970b-3c8f6e29ece2R01